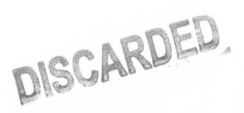

ALLERGIC
to the Twentieth Century

ALLERGIC
to the Twentieth Century

The Explosion in Environmental Allergies —
From Sick Buildings to Multiple Chemical Sensitivity

PETER RADETSKY

LITTLE, BROWN AND COMPANY

Boston New York Toronto London

First Edition

Library of Congress Cataloging-in-Publication Data

Radetsky, Peter.
    Allergic to the twentieth century / Peter Radetsky. — 1st ed.
      p. cm.
    Includes bibliographical references and index.
    ISBN 0-316-73221-4
    1. Allergy.   2. Environmentally induced diseases.   3. Toxicology.
  I. Title.
  RC585.R275 1997
  616.97 — dc21   96-40192

10 9 8 7 6 5 4 3 2 1

MV-NY

Published simultaneously in Canada by Little, Brown & Company (Canada) Limited
Printed in the United States of America

For Nancy

For Sam, Jessica, and Sascha

And for little Justine

Acknowledgments

Thanks to the many people — scientists, physicians, patients and their families — who afforded me privileged glimpses into their lives. And thanks to those who reviewed the manuscript for accuracy. The book is better for their efforts.

Thanks to my agent, Kris Dahl, for sticking with this project. Thanks to Bill Phillips at Little, Brown for his unflagging support and patience, and to Amanda Murray for whipping the book into shape.

And, as usual and always, thanks to my family.

Contents

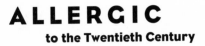

ALLERGIC

to the Twentieth Century

Allergic to the Twentieth Century

ON MY THIRTY-FIRST birthday I began sneezing. I had moved from the mountains of Colorado to the coast of California, and there, surrounded by a lushness of trees and plants unknown in the dry Rockies, I came down with what I thought was an endless cold. Sneezing and sniffing, eyes itching and nose dripping for months — this was my entrée into the world of allergies. Ever since, when the acacia trees bloom and grasses grow high, I reach for the handkerchief.

I'm not alone, of course. Over fifty million Americans suffer allergies. The statistical breakdown goes like this: Some thirty-five million people in this country endure the stuffiness and sneezing of hay fever — allergic rhinitis, as the allergists call it. It may be the single most common chronic disease experienced by human beings. Another fifteen million suffer asthma's constricted airways and difficulty breathing. Over four thousand die of the disease every year.

Less frequent allergies include reactions to insect stings and bites; pet dander (9 percent of Americans are allergic to cats); cockroaches and dust mites (inhaling the feces and dried skeletons of the insects is what causes the problem); medicines such as insulin, aspirin, and antibiotics; plants such as poison ivy. And molds and foods such as wheat, eggs, milk, fish and shellfish, and peanuts provoke reactions. Sometimes these allergens kill — some two thousand Americans a year die of allergy-induced anaphylactic shock. One out of nine trips to a doctor involves allergies, including one of every five visits to a pediatrician. Americans spend over $5 billion a year to cope with allergic disease.

I do my share. In an attempt to rid myself of my hay fever, I've been through the fiendish experience of an allergy test, in which dollops of allergens were dripped into tiny rents in my skin to see if they would provoke swelling and itching. It's something like stepping into a swarm of mosquitoes without being able to swat back. I've reclined almost naked on a padded table while acupuncture needles were tapped into my flesh in an attempt to stem the sneezing. I habitually load up the medicine chest with antihistamines and decongestants. But nothing really helps. Not in the long term, anyway. One thing allergy sufferers know all too well: like the tax collector, allergies always return.

But no matter how many boxes of tissue I plow through, no matter how miserable I become, no matter how much I complain, I know that compared to others, I have it easy. In fact, compared to others, I have absolutely nothing to complain about. For example, consider the sad story of Helen Keplinger.

A lawyer for the Environmental Protection Agency (EPA) since 1979, Keplinger first noticed her health deteriorating in 1985. The cause? As far as Keplinger is concerned, it was the very building where she worked. She feels she was poisoned by a sick building.

The term "sick building syndrome" is relatively new, coined in the early 1980s by occupational medicine specialists to describe the kinds of workplace illnesses that seem to have no other cause. The most famous example of the syndrome occurred right under the EPA's nose, at Waterside Mall, its Washington, D.C., headquarters. For some time employees had complained about the air quality in the building (reasons for the problem included an outdated heating, ventilation, and air-conditioning, or HVAC, system and overcrowding), but things didn't come to a head until 1987 and 1988, when the building was remodeled and 27,000 square feet of new carpeting was installed. Suddenly hundreds of employees became sick. One of those people was Helen Keplinger.

"When I moved into Waterside Mall in 1985, my office had been freshly painted, with new drapes and new carpet," she recalls. "Almost from the first day there, my mouth always had a bad taste in it. A metallic taste. I kept rolls of Lifesavers and chewing gum in my desk and ate them constantly because of that taste in my mouth. I also had a headache nearly every day, and I began to keep giant-sized bottles of aspirin and Tylenol in my desk. Most of the secretaries also had frequent headaches and came to my office for an aspirin."

Keplinger's health deteriorated rapidly. She began to have problems with her ears when she flew — and she was flying to Chicago on business once a month. And on Mondays, after a weekend away from the office, she began losing her voice. "Believe it or not," she says, "I rationalized that the problem was that I spent so much time on the phone, and this talking caused my voice to become hoarse — as if to say that I didn't use my voice at home over the weekend."

In 1987, her office was recarpeted, and her problems grew worse. She began to have severe headaches. She was constantly tired. A regular jogger for years, now she could hardly run at all. When she lay down to do back exercises, she became dizzy. She began forgetting things — the names of people she interviewed for jobs, the names of guests at a party, work documents, appointments, where she parked her car, phone numbers, even how to get to places where she was driving. She saw her first physician during this time. He had no suggestions.

In August of 1988, Keplinger returned to work from a week's vacation to find that her office had been painted again. "The next day when I awoke, my eyes were so red and swollen that I could barely see," she says. She went to a dermatologist. He assumed an allergic reaction, although Keplinger had no history of allergy. He suggested no tests, wasn't interested in hearing about her office, simply prescribed cortisone cream, and sent her on her way.

During the fall of the next year, 1989, Keplinger and her family moved to a new house, and they began to spend their weekends painting the walls. Meanwhile, Waterside Mall was being reroofed, painted, and wallpapered. Soon Keplinger could no longer stand paint at all. She became nauseated driving behind buses or riding inside them. She couldn't stand to be near people wearing perfume. Her life was becoming intolerable. "I found myself having recurring dreams of smothering," she says. "I started having nosebleeds and a twitching in my left eye."

Finally, in 1990, she asked her supervisor if she could work at home for a few days. "I had been sick with a recurrent respiratory infection for six months. I had taken three different antibiotics and I was no better. I could no longer stand to pump gas for my car, walk through the detergent aisle at the supermarket, or read the newspaper. Fabric stores made me sick, malls made me sick, there was almost no place where I found any relief." On the strength of a letter from Keplinger's family physician suggesting that she was suffering from something relating to her building, the supervisor agreed. She could work at home.

Today Keplinger is "coping." "As long as I work at home, avoid rush-hour driving, stay away from people wearing perfume in close spaces, avoid buildings where the indoor air problem is obvious when I enter it, then I am able to function well enough to do my job. The difficult thing is, of course, coping under these circumstance leads to extreme isolation . . ."

As for Waterside Mall, eventually the new carpet was removed and the HVAC system improved, with janitor closets and copy centers isolated from the main ventilation system — at a cost of over $4 million. The EPA is slowly moving offices out of the building. Approximately seventy-five people have been granted "work at home" status because of chemical sensitivity that every one of them attributes to the building's bad air.

Helen Keplinger has no illusions as to the seriousness of her problem. "Many of my professional colleagues think something has happened to me, but I don't think they understand what, and they don't ask. They understand that I work at home, but I don't think even the people in my immediate office understand what life is like for me. It is fair to say, I don't think my life will ever be the same."

Neither will Rick Kiessig's. "It was eight years ago," he says. "We were living in Mountain View at the time, and we had lots of rosebushes."

Kiessig is now thirty-seven years old. Large and thick, with pasty skin that looks as though it never sees the sun, Kiessig is a computer software consultant; and the California town of Mountain View is one of many that bead along the peninsula south of San Francisco, separated from one another by a mapmaker's dotted lines rather than any natural boundary. On a good day, a day blessedly free of haze and smog, it looks out onto the stark brown landscape of the Diablo Mountains — thus the picturesque name. But there's nothing picturesque about the town. Wide asphalt boulevards, relentless traffic, blank-faced buildings and shopping malls, franchise restaurants and electronic superstores — Mountain View lies in the heart of Silicon Valley. Kiessig and his wife, Lynne, now thirty-nine, had married only nine months earlier. They were just beginning to build a life together. He owned his own consulting business, she was pregnant — with twins, no less — and they had recently purchased their own home. The future looked promising, inviting, safe.

All that was about to change.

"I decided to dust the rose garden with a pesticide powder, an organophosphate, that you mix in the dirt around the roses," Kiessig recalls. "Well, our dog decided that he liked the taste of the stuff. He went around and ate a bunch of it.

"Then he came inside, got sick, had diarrhea, and threw up. All over the carpet in the family room. He then proceeded to *really* get sick. He couldn't even walk. I took the dog to the vet in an attempt to save his life. They were successful in the short term, but not in the long term."

"He did live, but barely," adds Lynne. "His nervous system was pretty well destroyed. We had to put him down two years later."

"Meanwhile," says Kiessig, "against my better judgment Lynne cleaned up the mess — with her bare hands."

"I used newspaper and towels," says Lynne. "But it didn't seem that they were soaking up *that* much . . ." Then she adds quietly, "Organophosphates are absorbed through the skin."

"That room was the main room we hung out in," says Kiessig. "We had the rug professionally cleaned the next day, but . . ."

No one knows for sure what happened, but something terrible befell Rick and Lynne Kiessig. Whether because of the rose-pesticide exposure or because of what Kiessig describes as "a long series of exposures to everyday chemicals and allergens," today the world is for them a hostile place. As with Helen Keplinger, substances in the environment that most of us take for granted, that we encounter daily without batting an eye, often without even being aware of them, make their life hellish. The short list includes chemicals like formaldehyde and chemical products such as pesticides, solvents, food coloring, and perfumes. Molds drive them crazy. Certain foods are virtually intolerable.

Rick is hardest hit. For him, the consequences of exposure to these substances range from "brain fog" — fatigue and inability to think — to partial paralysis, to being rendered virtually unconscious. He suffers from numb spots in his back, skin rashes, ringing in his ears, stomachaches, leg cramps, heart palpitations, difficulty sleeping.

"I made a bad mistake right about the time we moved out of our Mountain View house," recalls Kiessig. "I knew better, but I had parts of the house repainted. I got so sick I couldn't walk — Lynn had to help me out to the car. I couldn't talk. I could think — my head was clear — but I couldn't make the words come out.

"I'm also very sensitive to perfume. I think people must have this vision that perfume is made from flowers — this wonderful organic thing, back to nature and all that. They don't realize that perfume is made of chemical solvents that happen to smell good. They don't realize how damaging this stuff is."

Foods such as nuts and soy products also make Kiessig miserable. And molds are even worse. "My biggest problem is with molds. I'll never forget one of the first times I was tested for a bunch of molds. I was so completely out of it I could hardly talk."

Such symptoms didn't appear all at once, however. Rather they snuck up on Kiessig. "It was a bouncy road to the bottom," he says. "Symptoms came on slowly, and eventually I fell off the cliff," he says. When he fell, in the fall of 1993, he fell hard. He couldn't work, couldn't lead a normal life, couldn't do much of anything. It's only been since the beginning of 1995 that he has been able to get back on the job.

"I still can't be at work too long," he says. "I have a specially prepared office, with an air filter in it. I try to stay in there, try not to go out to the copy machine. But if I get a whiff of the copy machine, or of solvents, I have a tough time. Luckily, my employer understands and tries to make my life as comfortable as possible."

Lynne suffers similar miseries — but with one special added agony. As she was pregnant when she cleaned up the dog's mess, her exposure seems to have affected their kids. "They were about thirty weeks old gestationally when it happened," says Lynne. "It took us a while to figure out the connection."

The twin boys, William and Edward, were born with lung problems severe enough to require weeks of intensive care. Today both boys are as sensitive to their environment as are their parents. William especially. "He'll be laughing, happy, wonderful one minute," says Kiessig, "and then he eats some food, or touches or smells something, and suddenly he's crazy, throwing glass bottles, jumping around, screaming, just miserable."

"It's been a real roller coaster," says Lynne. "And people don't have much sympathy."

What happened to the Kiessigs? Did the blast of rose pesticide coupled with their other exposures destroy their defenses against the outside world? What happened to Helen Keplinger? Did her "sick building" make her ultrasensitive to common substances in the environment? Have they become, in effect, allergic to the twentieth century? No one knows for sure. But theories abound. One of the most persuasive suggests that what happened to them constitutes a new kind of disease, a disease brought on by exposure to irritants followed by a loss of tolerance to other, previously bearable, substances in the environment. In other words, specific exposures lead to a general intolerance. The name proposed for this theory is "Toxin-Induced Loss of Tolerance," or TILT. More often than not the initial irritant — or incitant — tends to be a product, or by-product, of modern industry. Often it may be a very low level of exposure. And, as with my suddenly coming down with hay fever at age thirty-one, it may well happen to anyone at any time.

Keplinger and the Kiessigs are not alone. You can hear stories like theirs all across the country. Some people, with similar exposures and similar sensitivities, cope better; some are even more devastated. Most people react most severely to chemicals, some to foods, some to invisible irritants such as electromagnetic radiation. Some may not even be aware of the source of their problems. But the common thread is a life altered by heightened sensitivity to substances in the environment that most of us take for granted, a heightened sensitivity almost always prompted by exposure to the commonplace products of modern living.

All of which leads to a real fix — how do you adjust your life so that you never come into contact with chemicals and other staples of everyday life? How, that is, short of taking off for the pristine mountains or desert or living in a cocoon? Perfume, for example. Good luck stepping onto a bus or train, or spending a day at the office, or entering any public place without encountering perfume. How do you avoid formaldehyde? Anyone who's ever taken high school biology recognizes the strong odor of formaldehyde. It is best known as an embalming fluid, but this omnipresent chemical is found in hundreds of products. Cosmetics, drugs, insulation, paper, particle board, permanent-press fabrics, plywood, preservatives — what they all have in common is formaldehyde. Want to avoid food coloring? Better stay away from oranges, sweet potatoes, Irish potatoes, soft drinks, cheese, butter, margarine, hot dogs, bologna, ice cream, sherbet, candy, Jell-O, maraschino cherries and other colored fruit, cookie and pie frostings and fillings, to name just a few. Pesticides? Not only do many people routinely treat their homes with pesticides, and not only are apartment houses often saturated with pesticides, but most of the commercially produced fruits and vegetables in the United States are sprayed with pesticides. Washing the food may not remove the residue. Solvents? Solvents are a prime component of paint and paint remover, varnish, ink, cleaning fluids, and such synthetic fabrics as nylon. The fact is that these chemicals are omnipresent, simply next to impossible to avoid. Reactions to such chemicals, therefore, could at the least alter, and at the worst destroy, a normal life.

Which is precisely the point. This degree of hypersensitivity can, and does, alter and destroy lives. Estimates of just how many lives are hard to come by. The National Academy of Sciences has suggested that some 15 percent of Americans may experience "increased allergic sensitivity" to chemicals. The extent of that sensitivity is not spelled out, but the number boggles — 15 percent of the population is over thirty-seven million people. Other studies suggest that the problem may be even more widespread. A 1991 survey by the U.S. Environmental Protection Agency found that approximately one-third of inhabitants of sealed buildings reported sensitivity to one or more common chemicals. In another survey, this one of the general population, 33 percent of 1,027 people reported chemical sensitivity. At the University of Arizona, college students were asked to describe their reaction to five common environmental chemicals: pesticides, automobile exhaust, paint, chemicals used in new carpets, and perfume. Sixty-six percent of them said that one or more of the chemicals made them ill; 15 percent pointed to at least four of the chemicals. When retired people between the ages of sixty and ninety were posed similar questions they gave similar answers. Fifty-seven percent reported that at least one of the chemicals made them ill; 17 percent implicated at least four of the five. Extrapolate those percentages to a U.S. population of some 250 million people, and the numbers are staggering.

The crux, however, is the severity and breadth of the reactions. If close to forty million Americans may experience some degree of chemical sensitivity, how many react like Rick Kiessig or Helen Keplinger? They are knocked out by their sensitivities; most of the people in these studies are not. Kiessig and Keplinger suffer a broad range of overlapping symptoms; the people in the studies react in more specific, discrete fashion. So how many might fit into Kiessig's and Keplinger's shoes? Nobody knows. But what everyone does agree on is that the numbers seem to be rising. And that, as with conventional allergies, the illness may well strike anyone, anytime.

This collection of miseries goes by many names: universal allergy, total allergy syndrome, allergic toxemia, cerebral allergy, environmental illness (EI), ecological illness, chemical hypersensitivity syndrome, chemophobia, immune system disregulation, multiple symptom complex, environmental maladaptation syndrome, chemical AIDS, twentieth-century disease — and there are more.

The tag that has caught on, however, is "multiple chemical sensitivity," or MCS. The people who often treat MCS sufferers, environmental physicians or clinical ecologists, define the problem this way: "Ecologic illness [MCS] is a chronic multisystem disorder, usually polysymptomatic, caused by adverse reactions to environmental incitants, modified by individual susceptibility and specific adaptation. The incitants are present in air, water, food, drugs, and our habitat." In other words, MCS is an adverse reaction to chemicals in our air, food, and water at levels that are generally accepted as safe.

This reaction can arise from chronic exposure to chemicals over a long time or from one huge dose. It can follow an infection, an auto accident, even giving birth to a child. And, after the initial onset, a strange spreading phenomenon takes place,

in which people start to experience reactions to other substances — other chemicals, foods, classical allergens. Keplinger's and the Kiessigs' increasing inability to tolerate just about
anything in the environment is a perfect example.

The keys are that the problem is chronic (once you have it
you tend to keep having it); it strikes more than one organ system; and the symptoms are many and varied. The likelihood of
coming down with it is influenced by your personal — most
likely genetic — makeup. And the provocateurs — the incitants — are everywhere, "in air, water, food, drugs, and our
habitat." For all intents and purposes, Keplinger, the Kiessigs,
and their compatriots are allergic to the twentieth century.

There may be good reason. Since World War II the use of
chemically based products and pesticides has increased expo-
nentially. New clothing, new carpeting, cleaning products, cosmetics, computer printers, copy machines, mothballs, particle
board, plywood, pesticides, perfumes, deodorizers, cigarettes,
food preservatives, vehicles, paint — the list of products that
incorporate and exude synthetic chemicals goes on and on.
And our increasingly tightly constructed buildings do a terrific job of trapping these chemicals and keeping them inside,
where a population that increasingly lives indoors can encounter them — thus sick building syndrome. New office buildings,
with their central heating and air conditioning and sealed windows, have been likened to upright airtight submarines. Even
the air inside the average American home can contain up to
150 different chemicals from household products and other
sources. Environmental Protection Agency studies of American homes indicate chemical levels two to five times higher
indoors than outdoors. Energy-efficient office buildings can
trap hundreds of hazardous substances, including dozens of
carcinogens.

Most chemically sensitive people do not suffer the extremes
of MCS, however. And they do not share Rick Kiessig's gender.
The profile of a typical MCS patient is white, thirty to fifty-

nine years old, a middle- to upper-middle-class professional, and female — just like Helen Keplinger. Some 80 percent of MCS sufferers are women. The vast majority of chemically sensitive people most likely experience relatively mild difficulties — headaches, fatigue, rashes — perhaps without even realizing their cause. Sneezing while walking down the detergent aisle at the grocery store is a common example of mild chemical sensitivity. Feeling a headache come on after sniffing perfume or cologne is another. Itchy eyes or stuffy nose from swimming in a chlorinated pool, nausea from inhaling car exhaust, and fatigue or dizziness after being exposed to a new carpet are others. I recognize all of them in myself. These relatively benign reactions pale when compared to the severity and breadth of the miseries experienced by people with MCS — but here's the rub: severe MCS may be the last stage of a continuum. What starts gently, almost imperceptibly, may end up as the full-blown horror of multiple chemical sensitivity.

If MCS is real, that is. *If* Helen Keplinger and Rick Kiessig and who knows how many others are truly suffering a debilitating new disease. The majority of the medical community doubt that. "Based on a lack of solid scientific data, the Council on Scientific Affairs of the American Medical Association cannot affirm that multiple chemical sensitivity syndrome (MCSS) exists as a recognized clinical entity." So states the *Journal of the American Medical Association.*

The reasons? They're threefold. In the first place, there are just too many, and too many kinds of, symptoms associated with MCS. Depression, fatigue, irritability, difficulty in breathing, headaches, insomnia, irregular heartbeats and other cardiovascular problems, paralysis, memory loss, upset stomach, conventional allergy-like problems such as asthma and hay fever, rashes, "brain fog" — what single disease could manifest itself in so many ways? An old saw in medical circles is that the more numerous the symptoms, the less credible the patient. Secondly, there are no reliable physiological markers for MCS. No widely accepted evidence that people with the disease consistently display a raised level of antibodies, say, or a proliferation of white blood cells — the kinds of signs that mark other diseases, including conventional allergies. And finally, the purported connection between MCS and exposure to common environmental chemicals has never been confirmed to everyone's satisfaction. As far as the medical establishment is concerned, horror stories such as Kiessig's and Keplinger's are just that — stories. The result is widespread skepticism concerning the validity of the disease. MCS is a disease without portfolio.

If MCS doesn't exist, then, where does that leave Rick Kiessig and his family? Where does that leave Helen Keplinger? Where does that leave the thousands — millions? — of others who claim at least some degree of chemical sensitivity? Where does that leave the very concept of a disease called Multiple Chemical Sensitivity?

Two possibilities. One is that, in the words of veteran National Institute of Allergy and Infectious Disease (NIAID) allergist Sheldon Cohen, "You're not dealing with a single entity. On analysis they're really a mixed group of people. Some are quite obviously a psychosomatic expression — some even may be off the deeper end. Some have organic disease, undefined. Some are really allergic — they fulfill the definition." In other words, these people may be suffering an assortment of problems, with various causes, that, while conveniently stuffed under the umbrella of MCS, do not constitute one disease and cannot be treated as such. And any approach that does so is barking up the wrong tree.

That's the more charitable possibility. The other is the likelihood that Cohen raises, and that most MCS sufferers have heard all too often and simply *can't stand:* perhaps the problem is psychosomatic — or, in the preferred term, "psychogenic." Perhaps their problem is all in their heads.

It's an understandable point of view. MCS-like symptoms are a hallmark of psychogenic problems. They even suggest hypochondria — as who does not know people who are always complaining of afflictions that seem to defy common sense? It comes down to that in the end: MCS just doesn't smack of common sense.

Yet it's been solidly established by now, a hundred years since Freud began to investigate the strange and powerful recesses of the mind, that the division between body and mind is an arbitrary one, and that "all in your head" has as little meaning as "all in your body." The mind and body are intricately interrelated. "Physiological" problems may have "psychological" origins — "psychological" problems may be "physiological" in nature. We treat "psychological" diseases such as depression, schizophrenia, and manic depression with drugs that affect the body; we use mind-related techniques such as biofeedback, meditation, and visualization to treat "physiological" injuries and diseases such as cancer. The line between mind and body has become irrevocably blurred.

So it's not surprising that any disease, MCS included, might have a psychological component. That is, if MCS is really and truly a disease. That is, if MCS exists at all. There is precedence for such skepticism with ill-defined problems. Chronic fatigue syndrome (CFS) and premenstrual syndrome (PMS), two maladies with similarly varied symptoms and similarly shadowy origins, were similarly impugned in their early days. Today few physicians dispute that PMS, anyhow, is a real problem. CFS, while seemingly on its own way to medical respectability, still provokes doubt. So while Helen Keplinger and Rick Kiessig are all too certain that MCS is a real and serious problem — their broken lives are proof — for much of the rest of the world, and much of the medical community, there's an enormous amount of suspicion. That's the uncomfortable place MCS sufferers find themselves: caught between a debilitating affliction and a world that more likely than not denies the very existence of their problem. "All in their heads," indeed. Are these people simply unfortunate, or are they crazy? They have been called both.

Or are they something else? Remember that people with MCS claim that their miseries are caused by exposure to common environmental substances, substances that most of us encounter every day of our lives. Perfume, building materials, food coloring, pesticides, paint, automobile exhaust, solvents, natural gas, detergents, bleach — these are as familiar to most of us as sunshine and as hard to avoid. Yet most of us are not laid low by such exposure. Why are MCS sufferers?

The answer, according to many of these people, is that they are, in effect, advance scouts, providing a warning of what might happen to the rest of us if we don't watch out. Against their will, simply because of their unwanted susceptibilities, they function as prophets, by their example crying doom for a society in which industry, with its essential chemicals and toxic byproducts, is in the driver's seat. In this context, the ongoing arguments about "all in the head" or "all in the body," about whether MCS is one disease or many, about whether MCS is real or not, fade. In this context the bizarre phenomenon of MCS is a call to action. What this mind-boggling affliction may be telling us is, "Look out!"

Chapter 1

Survival Strategies in a Hostile World

TODAY SUE PITMAN is fifty-two years old. In 1977, healthy and happy, she, her husband, and their two small children moved to a suburb of Chicago called Lake Bluff. Their house was located in a quiet neighborhood one block from Lake Michigan. It was brand-new. It seemed perfect. It wasn't.

During the first winter there, Pitman began suffering headaches. Then came a string of respiratory ailments, including asthma and pneumonia. Soon her kids — one-year-old son, Kyle, and daughter, Gwin, five — were plagued with ear infections, sore throats, depression. "We were sick all the time," she says. "We were constantly going to doctors, but nothing they prescribed worked."

By the second winter, Pitman and the kids were diagnosed with food allergies and allergies to dust and mold. Pitman herself began to suffer nausea, rashes, bloody noses, and bladder and vaginal infections. "I don't even remember all the symptoms," Pitman says. "They just hit us everywhere. The fatigue. Horrible, horrible, horrible headaches. The children's ear infections. Everybody having a sore throat all the time. Urinary problems." It was a nightmare.

For everyone, that is, except Pitman's husband, Lockett, an IBM sales manager. He seemed immune to the health problems bedeviling his wife and kids. Although no one realized it at the time, his continued good health was a hint as to the origin of their miseries — as were some surprising insights Pitman was starting to come up with.

"I found a book that showed how to test for food allergies by taking your pulse. I went through a period where I was testing pulses all the time. Once I grew some broccoli in my garden without using pesticides and tested that against broccoli that I got at the store. The commercial broccoli caused a change in my pulse; the homegrown broccoli didn't do anything.

"Then I had another experience. One day I was walking downtown in our little village, and all of a sudden my pulse *really* started going. I thought, 'What's going on?' I looked around and didn't see anything except a lady across the street with a watering can sprinkling the rock garden in front of the pharmacy. When I went home, I calmed down. The next day I went back to the pharmacy and said to the lady, 'What were you doing?' Well, she was putting herbicide on the rock garden."

There was one more clue: every time Pitman drove into the congested streets of Chicago to see a doctor she became ill. It was beginning to look as though exposure to chemicals, from herbicides to auto exhaust, played a role in her problems. So when in the fall of 1980 she happened onto a newspaper article about a local physician who specialized in the relationship between health and the environment, Pitman was ready to give him a chance. The doctor's name was Theron Randolph.

She didn't know it then, but Sue Pitman was about to embark upon an odyssey that would rescue her family — and change their lives. In so doing, she has become a heroine of the MCS community. For she has confronted the central question facing people saddled with the affliction: if you are allergic to the twentieth century, how can you survive in the twentieth century? The people we'll meet on these pages have tried various methods with various results.

Sue Pitman not only has survived, she has thrived. Sturdy and strong, with light brown, shoulder-length hair and striking blue-violet eyes, she could pass for an unexceptional, preppy mom. She's not. She has been to the depths. How far she had fallen was never more clear than when Randolph started explaining what he had gleaned from a detailed history of her ailments, a battery of tests, and his own experience with such problems. Sue, he said, was allergic to natural gas, herbicides, pesticides, formaldehyde, alcohol, dust, and molds. She was allergic to ethanol, a byproduct of automobile exhaust. And she was allergic to various foods — milk, corn, wheat. When she brought her kids in to be tested, the results were similar. The Pitmans were a family of chemically sensitive people.

That was the first blow. The second was when Randolph identified the primary origin of their sufferings. Not random auto exhaust, not an occasional woman dumping herbicide on her garden. It was their home, their long-sought dream home.

How could that be? Now, only three years after they had moved in, the house was still almost brand-new. It was tightly constructed and energy-efficient, furnished with new carpet, vinyl wallpaper, and formica-faced kitchen and bathroom cabinets specially ordered by Pitman. All of which was precisely the problem. These furnishings, as well as the treated materials used in construction, were awash in the very chemicals that Randolph had identified as the cause of the Pitmans' troubles. And when the Pitmans weren't being exposed to chemicals inside the house, they were exposed to more chemicals outside. All that small-town beauty, the expanse of green lawns and majestic trees, didn't come for free.

"It was a heavily pesticided neighborhood," Pitman recalls. "There was mosquito-abatement spraying every three to five days that first summer. The stuff was just sucked into our house." The chemicals used were malathion and resmethrin, both nerve poisons (and both derivatives of the notorious nerve gas sarin).

In this new light, then, the fact that Pitman's husband, Lockett, was the only one in the family to escape the illnesses plaguing the rest took on new significance. Why wasn't he afflicted? Because *he wasn't exposed as much.*

"He was a workaholic and spent most of his time at the office, not at home," says Pitman. "With small children, I didn't get around that much. The kids and I were home all the time, on the floor, on the rug" — a prime source of formaldehyde and other chemicals.

The final blow was Randolph's advice concerning what to do about their contaminated home: either safeguard it in hopes of avoiding those substances that gave them trouble, or, if all else failed, move.

At first the Pitmans took the less drastic route. "I was excited that somebody had an idea what was wrong with us, but I didn't really believe it for another couple of years," Pitman recalls. Her skepticism was understandable. How could she and her kids be sensitive to so many common substances? It seemed to defy logic. "Still, I was doing the things he told me to do."

Those things included buying air filters for the bedrooms, cutting back on those foods to which they were allergic, eating organic foods generally, and ridding their home of chemical cleaning products. And Pitman attempted to do something about the pesticide spraying around their house. "I sent registered letters to all the pesticide companies that did business in our little square-mile community and asked them for prior notification of when they were going to spray. Some of them notified me, and some of them didn't."

But while the measures did indeed improve their health,

they didn't completely alleviate the family's problems. So finally the Pitmans threw in the towel and moved. Pitman laughs. "We decided, like other people who don't make good decisions, to move to another house. *But in the same community!*"

This house was older and less tightly constructed, with furnishings that also were older, so that presumably more of their synthetic chemicals had dispersed. "It did have a gas stove and gas hot-water heater," says Pitman. "We had those replaced with electric." To minimize their exposure to automobile exhaust, they sealed off the indoor entrance to the attached garage. And they converted their large, tiled bathroom into a sleeping "oasis."

"One day I had asthma so bad I could hardly breathe well enough to talk," remembers Pitman. "I panicked. I called Dr. Randolph. The nurse said, 'Take everything out of the bathroom, cover up the toilet with aluminum foil to block exposure to chlorine in the water, put your air filters in there, and take cotton bedding with you. Lie down on the floor, and I assure you you'll be able to breathe.'

"So I did — and I was."

And subsequently she took the kids into the bathroom oasis with her. "Gwin slept in the tub, and Kyle slept on the floor with me. Meanwhile we emptied out our extra bedroom and made that an oasis where we slept from then on.

"Things got better," she remembers. "We did pretty well. Our new house was closer to the lake, on a bigger property, in the midst of even bigger properties. So we didn't have as much neighborhood spraying. We could convince the mosquito-abatement people not to come down to our house.

"But you never knew what might happen. Every time the kids went to a birthday party, for example. Once Kyle came home from a party with a side of his body paralyzed. It was crazy. I'd panic. 'What was happening? Was it going to turn into something worse? What could we do about it?'"

And while the spraying problem wasn't quite so severe

around the Pitmans' house, the rest of Lake Bluff was being sprayed as usual. "Every day there were professional applicators applying pesticides in our little town," Pitman says. "Especially in the summer. How could I expect that we could stay away from that?"

The truth finally sank in. If the Pitmans were to have any chance of living healthy, normal lives, they'd have to leave their home once again. And this time they couldn't stay in the neighborhood. They'd have to find a new place, a place that was relatively free of the pesticides and other chemicals that continued to plague them in the Chicago suburbs.

"I was *determined* to get better," Pitman says. "I didn't think it was fair for my kids to grow up living that kind of terrible life. I wanted to go for a total cure. But my husband said, 'We can't make another mistake. We can't *afford* to make another mistake.'"

That meant careful research. By this time Pitman was in contact with other chemically sensitive people across the country. She sent out a survey asking for recommendations for safe areas in which to live. "One response was from a lady who said, 'I'm answering this survey as if I was still chemically sensitive.'" Pitman laughs. "'*As if I was still chemically sensitive.*' *Bingo!* That gave me hope."

The responses emphasized three places in the country. One was the Mt. Shasta region of northern California. Another was the little town of Portrero in the mountains east of San Diego. And the other was a Texas town called Wimberley.

"We knew we had to live off and separate, but we didn't want to be totally separate. We wanted someplace that was close enough to a city to allow my husband to work — so that we still had an income." Pitman laughs.

Of all the possibilities, Wimberley seemed best able to meet those qualifications. Located in the hardscrabble hill country of south-central Texas, the little town is home to some eight thousand residents, including at least a dozen people with severe MCS. It's about as close to an ideal setting for these folks as you can get. There's not much agriculture — the rocky land is ill suited for farming — and not much industry. Thus there's not much chemical pollution. The area is dotted with antique and craft shops — no pollution there. Neighbors are few and far between. That means little threat of contact with perfumes, aftershaves, deodorants, hair sprays, and polyesters. The college town of Austin with its organic food markets is thirty miles up the road, and Dallas and Dr. Bill Rea's Environmental Health Center is just a few hours north. MCS sufferers can gingerly venture into the hazards of modern civilization for their goods and services, then retreat to the safety of their hill-country homes. (Says Rea, who treats most of the Wimberley MCS patients: "Nontoxic communities — they're a marker of our times. People trying to get air they can breathe.") In the spring of 1984, Pitman and her kids went down to take a look.

"I met a lot of the chemically sensitive people that I had identified in my survey," Pitman says. "When we went back home, we started to think about how we could get back there. It's hard to get off your duff and make a move like that, especially when you have your whole family to take care of. But it was summer, and our lives were getting intolerable again. I was thinking we wouldn't survive another summer."

Then Pitman got a call from one of the chemically sensitive people she had met in Wimberley. "I understand you're going to come build down here. Would you like to rent my apartment while you're building?"

Pitman laughs. "Huh? I wasn't ready to move quite that fast. And I wanted to be sure. So I figured, okay, we'll come down, move into the apartment, see if being in Wimberley really helps. We moved in July of 1984. My husband stayed back in Chicago. By December he was down here with us. We never went back."

*   *   *

Lots of refugees to Wimberley have never gone back. They can't — they've come to escape the twentieth century. But the irony is that the twentieth century — at least its media — doesn't want to let them alone. Wimberley's MCS sufferers have been profiled in the pages of the *New York Times, Life, Health,* and *USA Weekend.* They have been featured on numerous TV programs, including the ABC newsmagazine *20/20.* They have even inspired a character on the series *Northern Exposure.* And no wonder. The lengths to which they've gone in hopes of regaining and sustaining their health are at once poignant, mind-boggling, even comical.

There's the middle-aged man who can't tolerate wearing anything except white cotton clothing. There's the old woman who orients herself according to electromagnetic waves. There's the middle-aged woman who lives in a porcelain-lined trailer, communicating with her family by loudspeaker, and the former psychologist who lives in a nontoxic aluminum shack. There's the mom who wraps a sheet around herself during excursions into the outside world as a shield against contamination. There are the others who kept a safe distance between themselves and the *20/20* reporter who came to interview them so as to avoid inhaling the scent of his cologne. These people are so eccentric they resemble cartoon characters rather than flesh-and-blood human beings. And the media emphasizes that aspect, creating figures of fun, comic relief, or simply objects of ridicule. All of this leads to the kind of callousness exhibited on the air by Barbara Walters, who, after watching the *20/20* segment, remarked to the reporter, "*I'd* sit next to you if you were wearing perfume."

When it comes to dealing with the media, Sue Pitman is an experienced pro. She has to be, because the Pitmans have built for themselves an unusual, photogenic dwelling that has garnered much attention — what might be called an MCS dream house. It consists of two log cabin–like structures united by one roof and enclosed by a huge screened-in rectangular deck some 90 feet long by 30 feet wide, set in the midst of ten acres of cedar and live oak. The house perches 10 feet off the ground on piers set into water-filled moats that keep fire ants and other bugs from crawling up and into the house. That way the Pitmans need no pesticides. The washer and dryer and the Pitmans' automobiles are relegated to a barn-style garage at the end of a path through the cedars, 100 yards away.

But the simple notion of a couple of little log cabins under a single roof misses the point of this structure by a long shot. In the first place, this is *some roof.* Made of pine and supported by massive hardwood beams, it juts rakishly upward 33 feet into the Texas sky. In the second place, each of the two self-enclosed pine-and-Colorado-spruce cabins includes a partial second story, or, as the Pitmans prefer, "loft," brightened by large skylights. For example, the cabin that includes the kitchen, bathroom, and living area (the "poison side," according to Sue) also features Lockett's home office upstairs (he works in Austin). The other cabin includes Sue and Lockett's bedroom, daughter Gwin's bedroom, an upstairs office for Sue, and an upstairs all-purpose room for son Kyle. It's the "safe side." "There isn't anything in this side of the house but cotton bedding and clothing," says Pitman.

Besides their utility, the two living spaces afford the Pitmans a change of pace. "One thing I learned by going into chemically sensitive people's houses, and the reason we built two houses, is that a real problem is breathing the same air all the time," says Pitman. "You're never going to get anything perfectly clean and nontoxic. So if you have two different air frames, you can go from one set of pollutants to another set of pollutants, and give your body a little bit of a rest."

These are just the indoor living spaces. When the south Texas weather allows — that is to say, most of the time — the family lives "outside," on the massive screened redwood deck that surrounds the two enclosed structures. Here the Pitmans have their primary, "outdoor" living room, dining room, and bedrooms nestled into corners of the deck. Only on the stormiest days do they push their beds inside. "The only time we ever come in is when the rain is horizontal," says Lockett.

This indoor/outdoor space is striking. Look up and you see a massive flying wing of a roof; look down and the deck spreads outward far enough and large enough to accommodate entire school classes for overnighters. And look outside through the screens and you see nothing but trees and space — no houses, no people, perhaps an occasional deer. "Everything's natural. I don't cut the grass." Lockett laughs. "This is the way people in Texas ought to live. We don't have enough water to live any other way."

So successful have been their house and their strategy of avoiding the toxic outside world that today Pitman and the kids are well enough to spend most of their time away from Wimberley. Gwin, now twenty-four, has graduated college and works in Austin. Kyle, twenty, goes to school in the east. And Pitman has her own antipesticide consulting business. She spends her days in a tiny office in Austin with the name "H/E Solutions, Inc. Knowledge & Products to Reduce Exposure to Pollutants" on the door. She does, that is, when she's not at the capital lobbying the Texas legislature for stricter laws controlling access to pesticides and other chemicals.

"Our health is much better," she says. "It's still not a hundred percent, and I don't know if it will ever be a hundred percent. It's hard to put it on a scale — you forget how bad the bad was. And you don't know how much of being better is because you've learned to follow a less toxic path in life. I probably wouldn't be anywhere near as well as I am and my kids wouldn't be if we didn't know how to naturally avoid things. It's just part of us."

The Pitmans keep an apartment in town and return to Wimberley only on weekends. Today, as they stroll along the path toward the barn to do laundry, Lockett spies a deer stealing silently through the cedars toward the big house.

"Hello," he calls. "Hello there! What are you up to?"

"We've had a lot of really good times here," Sue says.

Seventy-four-year-old Annabelle Brausieck has not been so lucky. After nine years in Wimberley, she's still searching for the right combination of housing and living that will help her get well.

A tall, slim woman with short, dark hair and a forthright manner, bundled this cold, drizzly November Sunday morning into a blue parka and white knit cap, she greets me at the door of her small white house with a firm handshake and a statement: "You're wearing perfume." The remark puzzles me. I've used no cologne, no aftershave, no hair spray. I'm wearing cotton clothes; nothing has been dry-cleaned. And still she smells perfume. Only later do I realize that the odor must have been from the shaving cream — *unscented* shaving cream — that I used some five hours earlier. Her remark impresses upon me how little it takes to pierce the veil of people with multiple chemical sensitivity — and how permeated with chemicals is my own everyday life.

Meanwhile, Brausieck has not budged from her doorway. "Go ahead," she says, finally, "stick your head in." Her house is simplicity itself. One rectangular room with white walls, tile floor, a wooden table and a few wrought iron chairs, an iron bedframe, a small upright organ against the wall, a computer monitor and keyboard, and a glass door that seals away a large television set and the computer itself. Steel cabinets and stainless steel counters punctuate the kitchen.

But Brausieck has trouble tolerating even these spare, antiseptic surroundings. "I've never really, truly lived in this house," she says. "When it's warm enough to leave the windows open I can spend time in here. I watch TV. But the house is not safe; that's why I can't live in it. That's why I'm outside so much of the time."

When, on the advice of Theron Randolph, Brausieck and her husband, Ed, first came to Wimberley, they built a garage with a small living area. Brausieck couldn't tolerate it. "I lasted a month in there," she says. "I became so ill. So we set up a cot for me to sleep on out here in the driveway. That was all right because there was no traffic then or cars. When all that started, I moved to the back of the house. I slept under the stars that whole first winter — except for two nights I slept in the car. I had a ukelele — a baritone, not the little one. I'd sit there and play and sing at the top of my voice. That's what got me through. I know what it's like to be a bag lady. But without a nice warm manhole cover to sleep on."

The next fall, before the main house was even finished, Brausieck moved her "bedroom" to the back porch. "It wasn't screened, but at least it was under cover. Things began to look up a little bit. My husband would fix my meals and bring them to the door. I'd sit on the doorstep and eat."

Five years ago the Brausiecks built a special sleeping room — a $13,500 porcelain cubicle in back of the house. She invites me to take a look, but only through the window. ("If I open it up, the dampness gets in there, and the molds are really hard for me.") It's tiny — 6 feet by 9 feet by 8 feet high, just large enough for a bed. An air-filtering system pumps air in and out of the room. ("If I were to do it again, I would make it larger. There's not enough air in there — it gets very stagnant.") As the walls, floor, and ceiling are porcelain, one of the safest materials for chemically sensitive people, there should be nothing in the room to bother Brausieck. At least that was the idea. She couldn't tolerate that room either.

So for the past two years Brausieck has been sleeping on the back porch of her house — which is now screened-in at least. It consists of a concrete floor, a limestone wall, an aluminum roof, and screens on three sides. The view, over rolling hills, cedar, and live oak to a gentle valley ("here in Texas we call that a canyon," Brausieck says, laughing), is lovely. The only piece of furniture is an old iron bedframe, sandblasted to remove the last vestiges of paint. A galvanized iron trash can serves as a cabinet for bedding and clothing. ("I take my covers in in the daytime, dry them out, put them in the dryer," Brausieck says. "But when it's raining my bedding's pretty soggy.") Two library books lie pressed under a large rock on the concrete floor. "I had them standing on end for several days to let the chemicals outgas," she says. "But the moisture curls them. So I put a rock on them, and they straighten out again."

Usually Brausieck can handle books — at least that pleasure isn't denied her — albeit with special precautions. "I can read books if I put them out on the porch for a week, fan them out, get them all aired out. If I can't, I have a piece of Plexiglas that I put over the pages. At one time I had a reading box. I made one from a cake pan — put the book in it, put the Plexiglas on top. But I'm getting better — as long as the book isn't brandnew. I can read books that men give me better because men don't have perfume on their hands." She laughs.

Life comes down to this for severely chemically sensitive people. Special precautions for the most commonplace actions — the most ordinary situations fraught with danger unimaginable to those in the "outside" world. And here's where living in Wimberley offers compensations other than the view. It's a great comfort for MCS sufferers to associate with people who understand.

Not that the Wimberley population as a whole offers much in the way of understanding. This is the hill country of Texas, after all, an area of good ole boys, an area never known for welcoming outsiders, especially oddball outsiders. "People are becoming aware, but they're still very intolerant," Brausieck says. "They still call us crazy. Some of the tradespeople are nice though. Occasionally I'll go down to the Ace hardware store. I'll call ahead and tell them what I need. They'll bring it to the door. I'll pay them, and they'll bring me my change."

So Wimberley's MCS sufferers — at least some of them — band together. "From Austin on west we have a group of eight to ten of us that have become a family," Brausieck says. "We started a church a year ago. It's called the Jeremiah Project, because the prophet Jeremiah endured many hardships. Our pastor is a seminary student with MCS. She couldn't do her internship because she couldn't stand to go into churches to preach. She got permission from the seminary for our group to serve as her internship. It's an interdenominational church — she happens to be Presbyterian. We've started a singing group and choir."

"Are you building a church?" I ask.

"No," Brausieck answers. "When you have this illness, you're usually pretty poor. It's a beggaring illness. It takes everything that you have, everything you've built up. So we have no funds. We're trying to get grants, and there are a lot of people who contribute, even though they don't attend frequently. But we can't even support our pastor.

"We met here at my house for a while. We meet on people's porches. Once a month we meet out at Canyon Lake. I tried to get local churches interested, but they just couldn't understand it. They thought I was strange."

So Brausieck keeps on keeping on. Trying to understand what has happened to her, trying to feel better, trying to survive. "I have a great respect for the pioneers," she says. "Of course, many times they weren't ill. That's the hard part — the survival along with the illness."

And once in a while, in a life made narrow and desperate by a mysterious and relentless illness, she experiences an unaccustomed joy.

"A group of us who have this illness met for lunch at a restaurant in Austin," Brausieck says. "It has an outside pavilion, and they don't spray. We all had a grand time. I was high on the occasion. I stayed outside most of the time, but I was able to go in and get my food and bring it out. It was a wonderful feeling. It was so great. I was just bunny-hopping along."

She is silent for a moment, savoring the moment. "It was wonderful."

Rick Kiessig hasn't had many wonderful times lately, but he and his family hope to change all that. They've taken their lives into their own hands. They're trying to create for themselves a totally controlled environment by designing and building a "safe house" from scratch.

It's a warm July Saturday in the town of Los Altos, another of the communities strung along the peninsula south of San Francisco. The homes are typical upscale northern California — large and sprawling, with wood siding, lots of window, brick fireplaces, immaculate expanses of lawns and pine and carob trees. Except for this one. It gleams in the high sun, hard and metallic, sparkling like a jewel. Rick Kiessig's house, about halfway built, is made almost entirely of metal — steel framing, steel roof, aluminum siding. "He's trying to build a house with virtually no wood and no paint, which is a tall order," Paul Howe, Kiessig's contractor, tells me before I visit the site. "It's a pain, taking longer than we anticipated."

A tour of the house reveals just how much of a pain — and to what lengths Kiessig is going in a last-ditch attempt to make his life livable. The first indication comes even before we step inside. Parked at the curb is a small, porcelain-lined mobile home. It's Kiessig's home away from home, his retreat when he just can't tolerate the apartment he and his family are now renting. In the trailer, at least, he can get a night's sleep.

The half-finished house is spacious, 3,200 square feet of living room, family room, three bedrooms, two and a half baths, plus 800 square feet of detached garage — in total, 4,000 square feet of carefully controlled environment. The risky things the Kiessigs must contend with in the outside world — pesticides, perfume, formaldehyde, solvents, auto exhaust, molds, polluted air — will be blessedly absent from this home. This will be a sanctuary for them, the equivalent of a Wimberley retreat, a space station of sanity and health. At least, that's the idea.

As I walk through the place, it seems pretty clear that if any home can keep the dangers of the world at bay, this might be the one. It also becomes clear that this house is a personal statement, Rick Kiessig's rejoinder to a world that has dealt him and his family a bad hand. "He's been studying for a long time," Howe told me. "He finally got to the point where he thought he could design a house that's healthy for him."

In the first place, there's no wood. Wood can rot, and that means mold. Wood can be eaten by termites, which could necessitate pesticides. Soft woods give off chemicals called "terpenes," which the Kiessigs cannot tolerate. Eventually there will be a little wood, as doors will be slabs of solid hardwood, but now, with the house still a shell, framing and roofing exposed, there's none anywhere. It's an odd sight. Houses in the framing stage usually resemble a thicket of giant, upright wooden toothpicks girdled by an undergrowth of sawdust and scattered nails. Not this one. This is an Erector set of a house, not one single nail or speck of sawdust to be seen. Just naked metal struts, cross-supports, diagonals, and x-braces, surmounted by enormous horizontal beams of galvanized steel that support a roof of steel with baked-on forest-green paint. (And every one — *every one* — of these metal pieces had to be washed before it could be used, because the factory ships them in a thin coat of oil.) Rather than nails, what holds this house together is bolts and screws. An unbelievable number of bolts and screws. "There are a total of about *fifty thousand* screws in the house," says Kiessig with a shrug.

Another departure from normal building involves insulating the house. Because it might cause reactions in chemically sensitive people, normal paper- and foil-backed fiberglass insulation won't do. "We're using a special nontoxic insulation made of magnesium oxide," Kiessig says. "It's analogous to foamed concrete. They cover the interior wall with a metal screen, then shoot the insulation right through."

The windows in the house are double-pane, and all fixtures — lights and switches — will be tightly sealed away by special gaskets. The use of plastic, with its outgassing of chemicals, has been kept to a minimum. And, no matter that this is sunny California, the house has no skylights. "The architect wanted to put in skylights, but my wife and I resisted to the end," Kiessig says. "We've had bad experiences with skylights. They leak, which could invite mold growth."

Then a surprise: for such an expansive house, the three bedrooms are incongruously small. "You're in there unconscious for eight hours a day," Kiessig says. "So these rooms need to be especially clean. They need to be small — not enough room for clutter." In the kids' bedrooms the closet is freestanding, air circulating all around. "When a closet is behind closed doors, there's a tendency for clutter to accumulate, as well as a lack of air movement — which means mold growth, moths, the whole bit."

One other room stands out, a 12- by 16-foot area that Kiessig calls the "project room." "This is the only place we're going to allow any toxic-type things — if the kids want to paint, for instance," he says. The room can be completely closed off from the rest of the house. It will even be negatively pressurized — air from the rest of the house will flow into this room rather than air from this room flowing out. If toxic fumes accumulate there, they'll be pulled outside through the air-filtration system.

The house is entirely electric, except for the water heaters, which burn natural gas. These gas heaters, and their potentially toxic fumes, are housed in a small hut outside. The garage, big enough for three cars, also stands alone, separate from the house — no exhaust fumes will leak into the house from here. "We're putting in a vent and fan, so when you bring in your car you can crank the fan and blow the toxic fumes outside," Kiessig says. Connected to the garage, but accessible only from the outside, is a 3- by 3-foot cubby for storing paint, gas cans, and other toxic materials.

Landscaping will be simple. Since the family cannot tolerate grass, the dominant mode will be concrete driveways and walkways and low-allergy plants. "We'll have some trees — *bee-pollinated* trees," says Kiessig. And the family members will do their best to avoid the eucalyptus trees bordering the back of the yard. So far the pungent trees seem to be far enough away not to cause trouble.

Finally, the *coup de grâce*: the air-filtration system. "It's a highly technical ventilating system, a fantastic filtering-and-recovery system, the equivalent of a clean room in computer manufacturing," Howe told me. "The house is essentially airtight, so that all air that goes in and out of the system is filtered and controlled. Kiessig designed it with an engineer."

There it sits in a huge — 11 feet long, 5 feet wide, and 3 feet high — shiny, stainless steel box in the backyard. All the air that enters the house must pass through here. First it circulates through a cotton pre-filter, then into the guts of the system, 1,000 pounds of activated carbon blended with potassium permanganate, a purplish compound that culls out low-molecular-weight compounds like formaldehyde that may sneak past the carbon. Then the incoming air must navigate a cotton post-filter and finally a large industrial filter, which can remove particles as tiny as .3 microns in size. Thus purified and, if necessary, chilled by cooling coils, the air is piped inside by a brawny 3-horsepower motor. "This will make or break the house," declares Kiessig. "It's got to work."

If it doesn't . . . well, the Kiessigs don't want to think about their lives if it doesn't. The family is investing a great deal in this house. Money, certainly. "The cost has probably been about 30 percent more than a conventional house," Kiessig says. As a comparable conventional house might run $140 per square foot, already a handsome sum, 30 percent more represents a hefty burden. But money is only part of the investment. For the Kiessigs, this house represents the promise of a healthy life.

And for Kiessig, at least, the house represents even more. He's convinced that what he's doing is the wave of the future. "I don't think the medical community has caught up to the science in this area. It's clear that chemicals common in standard home construction are carcinogenic and immunotoxic. It may take a generation, but this is the way things have to move. When people discover that they're living in boxes that are toxic to them, they won't want to build the traditional way any longer."

Easy for him to say. Kiessig has a well-paying job. And his illness has not forced him to give it up. Not only has he been able to afford to build his own home, he has been able to afford the added expense of customizing it to his family's needs. And he has been able to afford the time to research "safe" home construction and design his own. Most MCS sufferers are not so lucky.

Take Lee Bloom, for example.

On a searing hot July morning in Tucson, Mark Sneller is on his way to rescue Lee Bloom. His trusty steed is a powder-blue '86 Toyota Supra, his weapons are in the trunk. They include a Flame Ionization Detector, a particle counter, and a miniature Roto-Rod particle collector. Sneller is about five foot, nine inches, broad-shouldered, athletic, with thinning light brown hair. He's a former karate teacher and, at fifty-five years old, a competitive masters swimmer with a rough-and-ready "don't mess with me" edge about him. He's also the founder and sole employee of the Pima County Office of Pollen and Mold and his own consulting firm, Aero-Allergen Research.

Sneller makes his living tracking down pollens, molds, and chemicals in a city that badly needs his services.

Remember when a cure for allergies was a retreat to the Southwest? One could be blessedly free of pollen and other allergens, because in the desert there were none. No ragweed, no freshly cut grasses, no pollinating trees, no mold. Just clean air, cactus, and sunshine. Cities like Tucson became virtual sanatoriums. In 1920, seven thousand of the city's twenty thousand residents had respiratory disease or allergies, with tent cities at the edge of town swelling with thousands more fresh-air pilgrims. Those days are gone. Since World War II Tucson has grown to become a bustling university metropolis of half a million people. The clean air also is gone. While Tucson has experienced a tenfold increase in population since the end of the war, its pollen has increased thirty-five-fold. Today fully *half* of Tucson's citizens, descendents of the original sneezing and snuffling squatters, have hay fever or asthma (compared to 15 to 20 percent in the U.S. population as a whole), and now they are living in a virtual downpour of allergens. Why? Because when allergy sufferers flocked from the East and Midwest, they brought along mementos from home: mulberry trees, olive trees, Bermuda grass. Today Tucson blooms.

"Decades ago we attracted people who had allergies, because it was a clean desert environment," explains Sneller as we drive through sun-drenched streets. "They came out and brought with them everything they ran away from. And their children have a hereditary disposition for allergies. So we have a higher percentage of the allergic population than most cities. It's incredibly ironic."

In response, Tucson has instituted allergy-relief laws, prohibiting the planting of pollen-producing trees, mandating that lawns be regularly cut, and introducing less offensive vegetation — all monitored by Sneller, who tilts at these windmills seven days a week, year round. A Ph.D. in microbiology and biochemistry, he is certified by the American Academy of Allergy and Immunology as one of its official national pollen and mold monitors. "The county contracts with me to run a number of pollen- and mold-monitoring stations for them," he says. "Basically I'm an independent businessman." He also consults for similarly besieged cities like Albuquerque, Las Vegas, and El Paso. "Let what we're going through be a lesson for everybody."

But pollens and molds comprise only part of Sneller's beat. He also tracks down toxic chemicals, and he is particularly wary of their effects in combination — their "synergistic" effects. A well-known example of the phenomenon is the mixing of barbiturates and alcohol. Taken by themselves they can be hazardous enough — in combination they can be deadly. Another involves radon and tobacco smoke. Radon, a radioactive gas, often shows up in homes and commercial buildings. Ordinarily it attaches to walls and furnishings, there to decay harmlessly. When there's smoke around, however, the gas particles tend to cling to fragments in the smoke and may be breathed deeply into the lungs. But the synergistic effects of most chemicals are simply not known. Sneller wrote his doctoral thesis on the impact of combinations of drugs on experimental animals. "It's real scary," he says. "The synergistic effects of chemicals are not measured, nor can they be measured. The potential damage of some of these compounds boggles the imagination."

This morning Sneller's rescue mission focuses on chemicals. Lee Bloom suffers from MCS. She also suffers from the lack of a permanent place to live. Sneller is going to test a prospective apartment to see if it's safe for her.

"Lee has been trying to find a place to live for years now," Sneller tells me. "We've monitored and measured, monitored and measured, and every time we think we've found something that's workable, there's always, always something that's not quite right."

Which, of course, is typical. "With chemically sensitive

people there's *always* some factor that isn't right," Sneller says. "And if it's a fragrance that bothers them, they're particularly out of luck. Perfumes are oil-based, and you just can't get them out. You can't shampoo them out, you can't vacuum them out, you can't scrub them or wash them out. If there's *any* smell around from perfume, then forget it — you might as well walk out the door and keep on looking."

We pull up to a nondescript cluster of some fifteen boxy, white stucco buildings arranged in rows separated by asphalt driveways. It looks like a motel court. Lots of driveway, lots of asphalt, lots of narrow, covered parking spaces, no trees, no grass, lots of sun. The complex lies barren and exposed in the 107° heat.

We knock at one of the units and step inside. It's small — living/dining room with fireplace, cramped kitchen, two bedrooms, a tiny patio just visible through sliding glass doors. Like almost everything in Tucson, it's air-conditioned.

There on the couch sits Lee Bloom. She's a tall, dark, attractive ex–New Yorker in her fifties dressed in a blue bathrobe. Her right arm quavers from Parkinson's disease. A desperate, pained look lights her eyes. Next to her sits Barbara Bleckman, whose house she has been sharing since March of '94. Barbara also suffers from MCS, and arthritis to boot — she wears braces on both wrists. She doesn't want to see Lee thrown out into the cold, but two years of camping in the living room of a 1,500-square-foot, one-bedroom house is a long time. Lee needs to find her own place.

"I'm an artist," Lee tells me. "I wasn't making much money from my art, but I had done okay in New York. Now here I am over fifty, and I'm sick." She presses a surgical mask to her nose and mouth. "I've never been allergic before. But I've found out that it is very common for women my age to develop MCS."

In Lee's case, as in so many others', the trigger seems to have been pesticides. "I had been on the waiting list for this subsidized housing situation," she says. "It was a place for disabled and elderly people who were eligible financially. I waited about a year and a half to get in there. It was a really nice apartment in a three-story building. It faced the football stadium, had sunset views, and was all electric.

"Then in March of 'ninety-four, a year after I moved in, they fogged the building with pesticides. They told us they were going to do it. They didn't tell us what they were going to use. But being a New Yorker, I never thought twice about pesticides."

Lee's voice breaks. "I'm getting a real bad headache in here." She presses the surgical mask to her face.

The apartment manager told Lee to clean out her kitchen and bathroom and leave for four hours. She went back that night, and, with Barbara's help, cleaned the apartment. Then she went to bed. "I hadn't made my bed that morning. I didn't realize they had done my bedroom too. When I got into bed, I got really sick. I was sleeping in the stuff. I thought I was having a heart attack. Barbara picked me up. She took me to the emergency room. They put me on a breathing machine. They said that I was suffering from inhalation exposure. They said not to go back to that environment.

"But where else was I supposed to go? I went back three times. I had friends in the building airing out the place, but it didn't help. By the third time, I had to leave after twenty minutes. I signed out of the building and went to live with Barbara." Lee breaks into tears. "If it weren't for Barbara, I'd be dead."

While Lee talks, Sneller stalks around the apartment with what looks like a Geiger counter strapped over his shoulder. This is his Flame Ionization Detector. Strapped to the bottom of the machine is a tank of hydrogen gas, which he lights — *whooosh* — before turning on the unit. The machine then pulls air through the flame, which ionizes the particles in the air and counts them. "I don't know anybody else who uses this. It's a piece of equipment I had my eye on for years. Cost me only four thousand bucks. I got a nice discount on that," he says, with independent-businessman pride. The machine spits and crackles as he moves from room to room.

His particle counter, a blocky boom box–like machine, stays put. Right now it rests on the counter near the kitchen sink, counting the particles in that room. It too pulls in air, but instead of shooting it through a flame, the counter passes the air through a laser beam. Every time a particle breaks the beam, the machine chalks it up.

And in every room — the living room, the kitchen, the bedrooms, the bathroom — Sneller has parked his miniature Roto-Rod particle collectors, small boxes with spinning propellers whose sticky arms snatch whatever may be floating through the air. Throughout the apartment the rotors whirr, tiny helicopters struggling to take off.

"What the particle counter does in toto, the particle collector does specifically," Sneller says. "It gathers the particles without burning or losing them. Then I can do the microscope work. If the counter says there are twenty thousand units passing through the laser beam, I can break down those twenty thousand units into this many molds, this many kinds of pollen, this much cigarette smoke, this much latex from auto tires, et cetera, et cetera. So I'm able to get a breakdown on what's happening in the building."

What's happening in this building is mixed news for Lee Bloom. First the good news: "Your total particle load is low — mold, pollen, plant parts, dust in general," Sneller announces. Then the bad: "But this place is loaded with perfume. And the first place it goes is into soft furnishings. Then it outgasses from the soft furnishings, including carpets and sofas. It can outgas for months, years, after the source is gone."

Desperate, Lee is undeterred. "Number one, the carpet would have to go, right? I'd have to replace it?"

"Yeah. That'd be the first thing. Just get it out of here. Don't shake it around. Roll it up and take it out carefully. Takes about an hour, and it's done."

"Any concern about the fireplace?" Barbara asks.

Sneller shakes his head. "The fireplace you can enclose in glass."

But by this time it hardly matters what he recommends. Lee's face and arms have broken out in red hives. Her headache is worse. In tears, she excuses herself and disappears outside. "The thing that's most disturbing about this illness," she says, as the door closes behind her, "is the high suicide rate. Just a tremendous suicide rate."

In the car on the way back to the office, Sneller explains: "Quite frankly, I'm at a loss why she called me on this one. We just walked out of an identical scenario, and now she's calling me again, same thing. The last one, I could hardly smell the perfume — this one, it's overpowering. Wouldn't bother you or me, though. We'd have it cleaned and call it a day."

He concentrates on driving for a few minutes. "People like Lee grasp at straws," he says finally. "She's desperate. She wants every place she sees. That's why with people like that it's hard to separate their psychological problems from their physical problems, because even a normal person would go nuts with that kind of running around."

"What can she do?" I ask.

"She can sign a lease if she wants, see if the management wants to take up the carpet. That's the only shot she's got. I'm gonna tell her, 'Here's the situation, Lee. Do what you want.'"

"What will she say to that?"

"She'll say, 'What's your recommendation?' I have to be honest. I'll say, 'My recommendation is, forget it.'"

But people with MCS can't forget it. They have to live *somewhere*. Not all of them can take off into the hills. And not all of them can build their own custom houses. Luckily for Lee, Barbara Bleckman provides her safe haven. Barbara has transformed her home into a place she and Lee can tolerate. She has totally gutted it, removed all carpeting, put down tile everywhere. She's sealed off all walls with forty-five gallons of nontoxic paint. And the house is in the foothills outside town, so it isn't exposed to traffic fumes and other city pollutants.

"Many other MCS people have been in my house and think it's one of the safest homes," Barbara says. "But everyone has to find a place safe for themselves. That's what we've been trying to do for Lee."

In Marin County, north of San Francisco, the search for a safe haven has resulted in a new apartment complex — the first, and only, such government-sponsored project aimed at MCS. The complex is the brainchild of Susan Molloy, a spirited forty-seven-year-old chemically sensitive woman who in 1988 was working as a volunteer at Marin Homes for Independent Living, an organization that owned and managed a housing complex for disabled people. Molloy fielded so many calls from MCS sufferers desperate for housing that she began to wonder whether it might be possible to build apartments that were not only safe but affordable. With Tom Wilson, president of Marin Homes, she began a four-year campaign to find a site, a contractor willing to work under severe guidelines and restrictions, and — most important — a way of funding the complex. "The hardest part of the project was conveying the idea to the greater community, both to the people who were instrumental in planning and funding and to ourselves," Molloy told the *Washington Post*. "We are so used to having to live this underground existence and not being treated in a legal sense as well as other people are treated."

In 1990 all that changed. The U.S. Department of Housing and Urban Development, flying in the face of the controversy over whether MCS was real or not, decided to recognize the disease as a disability. MCS sufferers therefore qualified for assistance. That's all the impetus Molloy and Wilson needed. They formed a coalition of nonprofit groups that included Marin Homes for Independent Living, the Ecumenical Association for Housing, and a support group for chemically sensitive people called the Environmental Health Network and set to work trying to convince HUD to help fund their project. And in 1990 HUD came through, to the tune of $1.2 million to build the complex and a promise to subsidize tenants' rents thereafter. Molloy's dream would actually become reality.

The reality has not been pleasant. The complex, called Ecology House, opened to MCS sufferers in the fall of 1994. Built on a corner lot in a residential area in the town of San Rafael, near San Francisco Bay, it consists of eleven units spread over two stories overlooking a central courtyard. From the street, with its green stucco, gray siding, patios, decks, and picture windows, the structure looks much like other apartments and town houses in the neighborhood. Look inside, however, and it's another story.

In the first place, that light gray siding may resemble wood, but on closer examination it reveals itself to be metal. Rap it and it vibrates. Same with the doors — they're metal too. Push one open and look inside an apartment, and you find a floor made of light brown tile held in place by grout of pure Portland cement with no additives or adhesives. Kitchen countertops gleam with shiny stainless steel rather than laminated plastic; kitchen cabinets are metal rather than wood, with baked-on white enamel surfaces. The stark white unsealed plaster walls conceal diagonal Douglas fir sheathing rather than plywood. And when plywood *was* used in construction, it was covered with foil so as to block the odor of its glues and formaldehyde. Window frames are aluminum sealed with silicone, which was judged safer than petroleum-based butyl caulking. Ceramic tile lines the window sills. And metal miniblinds rather than drapes fill the window spaces — they're easier to clean and won't attract mold.

The apartments are all electric — no gas and combustion odors to deal with — and are heated by hot-water radiators along the baseboards. Ceiling fans keep the air circulating.

Drinking water is filtered to remove chlorine. Bathroom fans vent to the roof, not to the sides of the building, so that any odors can be carried aloft by the sea breezes. And on the second floor a small screened-in area serves as an "airing room," a space where tenants can allow potentially bothersome stuff to outgas. All in all, each unit is a one-bedroom, 540-square-foot box of pristine, nontoxic space. And the complex's strict house rules mean to keep them that way. Among the restrictions: no pets, no smoking, no perfume, no cologne or aftershave, no scented lotions or shampoos, no paints, no glues, no burning of any substance, no idling of engines in the parking lot.

Nearly a hundred MCS sufferers applied for the complex's eleven apartments. Those who made it through the draw were offered a forty-eight-hour trial period without charge. And they were greeted by a disclaimer, in boldface: the Ecology House board could not "warrant or guarantee the safety of the materials for all persons with MCS/EI."

The disclaimer was prescient. Marta Sonnenblick's story is typical. A gray-haired nurse from Sweden who attributes her sensitivity and resulting neurological damage to a reaction to mercury in her dental fillings ("I'm fifty-eight, and I look like I'm sixty-eight," she laments), Marta was one of the first people to move into Ecology House. "I thought this was just fabulous — low rent, a safe place," she says in faintly Swedish-flavored English. (Rent *is* low, a sliding scale up to 30 percent of the tenants' income. They are allowed to make up to $21,000 a year and still qualify for occupancy, but most don't come anywhere close to that figure.) "I looked at it as a place where I would stay for a couple of years and get myself healthy. Then I would go out and resume life as a normal person."

It hasn't worked out that way. "From the beginning it smelled a little bit weird," Marta says. "The first night I tried to sleep, I slept for just two hours. Then I woke up and thought I was going to *die!* So many aches and pains. I was all swollen up."

Compared to the experience of other tenants, Marta's reaction was mild. Dorothy Robertson also detected an odor when she moved in and pushed her windows wide open for a few days. Then the weather grew cold, so one night she shut the windows and climbed into bed. Within an hour she was in anaphylactic shock. She crawled onto the patio, where she spent the night. Since then she has been staying with friends.

Jan Heard wore an oxygen mask in her apartment. Without it she suffered headaches, nausea, joint pains, and arthritis. She slept on a mattress supported by cinder blocks, reasoning that if she brought her own bed into the apartment it might absorb whatever it was that the place was emitting. In fact, like Robertson, she rarely stays at Ecology House any longer. "Everyone I've known with environmental illness who has visited me there has gotten sick within a half hour," she told a local newspaper.

And "Richard Underwood" ("That's the name I go by. It's not my legal name. I've got a chronic illness, and I don't want everyone to know who I am") has been sleeping either outside or in his bathroom. "I sealed myself in," he explains. "Taped up the door, made an air barrier between the bathroom and the rest of the apartment. And since the bathroom walls have a different composition, I was able to spend nights in there. I could keep on doing that. It's a tolerable space for me. But I'm awfully big, and I'd like to use it as a bathroom, which makes it less desirable as a bedroom, so . . ."

Richard *is* big, a gangling six feet, four inches. The thought of him curled up on the bathroom floor night after night would be comical if it weren't so sad. Also comical if it weren't so sad is his proposed solution to his troubles. "From my experience in the bathroom I've come to the conclusion that they've done only one thing wrong," he tells me. "The only substance they allowed in here that I have a problem with is the wallboard. You probably can't smell anything. But after I've been here a while I can detect a glue-like smell. Unfortunately, there's a thousand square feet of that particular substance in here. That makes it a big problem for me."

Richard knows it's the wallboard because he's tested the other possible culprits, the metal cabinets and doors. "I took all the painted metal surfaces out — kitchen cabinets, doors," he says. "I just finished putting them all back. It was an attempt to figure out if taking out the cabinets would significantly improve the quality of the indoor air for me. Sad to find that it didn't. I spent several weeks doing that experiment. Now I'm going to try another one."

This next experiment, Richard hopes, will make it possible for him to continue to live at Ecology House. "I'm going to construct, *indoors*, a garden shed made out of anodized steel. You can purchase these things for under three hundred dollars — that's cheap enough for me. I'll put it up in the bedroom, make that my vapor barrier between the walls and where I live. It'll be a room within a room." He thinks of the possibilities for a moment. "If it works, I could possibly put another one in the living room. But it might be a little silly to spend all that money . . ."

For Richard, money is the issue. He's not thrilled with Ecology House, doesn't even particularly like it, really. And he's not thrilled at the prospect of living in an indoor garden shed. But the housing complex offers him a place he can afford. He just can't pass that up without a fight. "I kind of feel a little embarrassed talking about this — here I am talking about, wow, what a great free lunch this is. But it's just that with my MCS I find it impossible to work. I haven't been employed in a significant manner in the last ten years. It's certainly one of the things that made me look very hard at this place. That's why I'm going through all these contortions seeing if there's any possible way of making this work for me."

The way Marta Sonnenblick has made Ecology House work for her — at least partially work — is by covering the walls in her apartment with plastic. For me, the effect is unsettling —

something like being inside a weather balloon, thick sheaths of translucent polyethylene masking bare white walls — but the starkness and sterility don't seem to bother her. Nor does the odor of the plastic itself, a common aggravation for chemically sensitive people. "It doesn't smell at all," she says. "It was a big job putting it up, but it's made the place so I can sort of manage."

There, in a small hardwood sofa, her back to the plastic-covered wall, Marta sits — wearily trying to make the best of a bad situation, wearily trying to survive. The thought of her, and the others struggling to ride out the problems at Ecology House, fills Susan Molloy with regret. But she needn't be surprised — the project has seemed star-crossed from the beginning. In fact, the most straightforward thing about it was securing funding in the first place — $1.2 million from HUD and an additional $600,000 from local sources.

"As far as HUD was concerned, this was just another disability. They funded the project out of their regular Section 8 programs for disability housing," says Katie Crecelius, a consultant specializing in low-income housing who has been closely involved in Ecology House from the beginning — and who does *not* suffer from MCS. "The Marin County community was *extremely* supportive. It wasn't easy to raise the money, but that was not nearly as hard as finding the site."

Ah, yes, the site. It presented the first roadblock.

"Katie and I looked for sites for three years," says Molloy. "We walked all over Marin and Sonoma counties looking at farmland and coastal property, remote areas with good air. Whenever we found anything good, we'd call friends with MCS and any kind of nontoxic-construction background, and a gang of twelve to twenty of us would descend on some site and sit there and see what was up. We'd see how we reacted to the site. People would say things like, 'Power lines are too close,' or 'There's a bog down there, but it looks doable,' or 'Pollen's driving me nuts, but I guess I can get an air filter.'

We didn't want to make a move without having some kind of consensus."

But despite all their effort, their search for a suitable site ended in failure. "All the places where we had a prayer, either HUD said it was untenable, or some aspect of funding fell through," Molloy recalls. "For one place on top of a lovely hill site in Novato, the farmer had to have all cash *right now*. And HUD can't pay people that way. Another place was really great. It was the site of a monastery, and they didn't believe in pesticides. People had been hand-carrying caterpillars off the forty acres for years. But it was on a hill, and they would have had to level almost the whole hill to get a gentle enough grade so we could follow HUD's rules to have wheelchair accessibility from the front door to the bus stop. No matter that there was no bus for fifty miles, and people with our cluster of disabilities are unlikely to go on a bus anyway."

Nor were the local powers any more flexible. "In Marin County all the wonderful open land is zoned for very low density," says Katie Crecelius. "It was made clear to us that there would be no changes, no compromises, no concessions. As far as the local politicians were concerned, you can't compromise even once because it sets a precedent."

Any compromising, then, would have to be on the part of Crecelius, Molloy, and Ecology House. Although for Molloy, when it comes to the final site, "compromise" is too weak a word. "The site is dreadful," she says. "It wasn't a choice. It was what we were left with after nothing else worked. Several of us hated it. We badly needed a rural site, but this site is congested. The power lines are too close for many of us, and it's in a neighborhood were there's no control over several thousand people. Any of them could light up their goddang hibachis at any moment. At the San Rafael city council meeting, when they said it was okay for us to be there, some doctor showed up in scrubs from the emergency room at Marin General and said, 'I live in that neighborhood, and I don't want these guys there. I have to deal with sick people all day, and I want to go home and relax and not have to protect these guys.' That made us swallow real hard. We thought, 'Oh, shoot, what if they all decide to spray-paint and drive us all out?' But it came down to that site or nothing. HUD had their hand on the plug. They wanted their money back *now*."

The adoption of the present site represents a crucial turning point in the story of Ecology House. It was then that the nature of the complex, its potential as a "safe house" for chemically sensitive people, became compromised. If any such project, ever, could be totally safe, this certainly wasn't going to be the one. "We cried," says Molloy. "We were pretty much despondent. Then we decided, the heck with it. If we can make a place where people aren't getting pesticided, and their neighbors aren't painting the walls all the time, and there's no carpet, then that might save some lives while people look for something better. We said, 'Let's change the name. Let's make it "Less Toxic Than Usual Apartment Complex" or something and drop the name "Ecology House," and try to lower people's expectations as much as we can.'"

But in that the Ecology House developers failed also. As they had to fail, given the desperation of MCS sufferers and their inclination to turn any glimmer of hope into a beacon. It's likely that nothing anyone might have said or done could have diminished the hopes surrounding the project. Says Molloy, "Expectations are still that it's going to be a red hot place to live. But it can't be — not in lowland San Rafael with power lines a couple of miles from the freeway."

And not when the building materials themselves may be intolerable. This is the second crucial breakdown in the disappointing history of Ecology House: whether because of ignorance, oversight, or the unfathomable difficulties of MCS itself, the physical structure seems to exacerbate the problem. Most of the tenants agree that the walls and cabinets are the primary offenders. Yet those are areas with which Katie Crecelius and her compatriots took special pains in an effort to accommodate MCS sufferers. The plaster covering the gypsum wallboard was purposely left unsealed, as it was feared that painting the plaster would prove more toxic than leaving it alone. "What's better, gyp board and paint or a plaster wall? Who knows?" laments Crecelius. And the metal cabinets with their baked-on enamel surfaces were judged to be the least toxic alternative. "Unless you're able to do all stainless steel cabinets, which would have been very, very expensive," says Crecelius. "I would have done that in a minute if I had had unlimited funds." The only trouble was, when the cabinets arrived, they reeked. "They did smell funny when they came in," Crecelius recalls. "We expected no smell, but they did have a smell. It wasn't as bad as painting a room, but they did have an odor."

Critics charge that the powers that be should have known better. And the reason they didn't know better was that they didn't rely on expert consultants during the planning process. Neither did they confer with physicians who treat MCS. Rather, the kind of testing most of the materials received was informal, to say the least. For example, take the plaster-covered wallboard: "We wanted to get something that would not be painted drywall, because we all intensely dislike painted drywall," recalls Susan Molloy. "Plastered drywall sounded like a good idea. People sent samples from all over the place, and lots and lots of us smelled samples and tasted samples and put them on our skin. And they seemed pretty doggone bearable. So even though it was more expensive than regular drywall, we thought that's the way we should go, so people wouldn't have to contend with paints."

Katie Crecelius defends this ad hoc approach. "One of the criticisms that has come out in the press is that we didn't consult any experts. What experts? Where are they? The body of scientific knowledge about MCS, such as it is, hasn't been pulled together in any kind of university or research institute, which is the traditional way we gather knowledge. During the design process, it was like walking on Jell-O. There was no firm ground anywhere. You just had to do something. So what we relied on a lot was anecdotal information from people with MCS."

For Molloy, however, neither the lack of a formal consultant nor this "touch, taste, smell" approach was the overriding problem — rather, it was the lack of quality control during construction. "What was needed more than a consultant was a cop," she says. "Somebody on site, with an *attitude*, who said, 'Hey, wait a minute, I think I can smell paint on those doggone cupboards — what's going on here?' There's no consultant in the world who would have camped there and done that job."

In fact, she says, the first shipment of cabinets *was* sent back to the manufacturer by the contractor in charge, because they were backed by wood. "And he took a lot of flak for that," Molloy says. "They reshipped him cabinets that were all metal but had some god-awful smelly paint on them. The contractor figured, 'Well, this must be the stuff the guys want, but it smells like paint.' And Tom Wilson said, 'It smells like paint.' Everybody who went in there said, 'Gee, these things smell of paint.' That would have been an ideal time for somebody to have said, 'Send them back!'"

But nobody did. Nor did anyone complain when the coat of plaster covering the drywall turned out to be much lighter than expected. "The plaster's extremely thin," says Molloy. "It's not the same wedding cake–frosting thickness that came on our little sample. It's kind of a skim coat. So even if the wallboard itself were tolerable, which is by no means necessarily true, there's not enough plaster over it to cover the stuff up."

So, the place needed a cop. Molloy regrets that she couldn't have played that role. For all her vision, she never lived at Ecology House. In fact, she never saw the complex completed, as she became too sick to stick around (she now lives in an Airstream trailer in rural Arizona). For that, she blames herself, and she kicks herself, because she could have been a darn good cop. "The cop should've been me," she says, "but I got real sick and had to move to the desert and couldn't perform my responsibilities. I wish I could've hung in there long enough. Maybe I could've gotten mad enough after the first couple of errors and gone ahead and chained myself to a grab bar or a banister and worn my respirator and sat there and monitored the construction. If I would've gone down in flames, it would've been worth it. I can't go back now. We needed that cop there — I couldn't keep myself together to do it."

But that was then; this is now. What can be done about Ecology House? Susan Molloy has an idea or two. "Whatever the screwups are, they're fixable. The walls can be sealed, with as nontoxic a sealant as possible. The cabinets could be covered with foil. I don't understand why somebody hasn't attacked Ecology House with several acres of aluminum foil. Or the bad stuff could be removed. Pull all the cupboards and cabinetry out of each unit, put them all out in the parking lot, apologize profusely to the manufacturer, and say, 'We'd like to have you pick these up. You can bake them properly, recoat them and paint them, sandblast them, or give us back stainless steel. But whatever kind of finish you guys put on these cupboards and closets is extremely, seriously problematic. We are not able to use it.'

"See if they'd make a deal on the basis of which kind of embarrassed they'd rather be. What would they like to be famous for? Their picture in the paper rejecting all these cupboards in the parking lot? Letting a bunch of guys get sick and having a bunch of guys like me go on television to say it's their fault — which I'm absolutely willing to do. Or do they want to be good guys and say, 'Oh, shoot, you're right, this isn't exactly what you ordered. Let us help you'?

"They screwed up. But even if they were just filling orders, knowing the nature of the project, I would think their customer-service guys would have said, 'Hey, isn't that the funny project in San Rafael? Don't we need to be careful?' I would love to get my hands on their board president."

But that will be hard to do from the Arizona desert. It's left to the Ecology House board and Katie Crecelius to actually deal with the problem. And Crecelius herself feels that for the most part their hands are tied. "With respect to the cabinets," she says, "it would be difficult to do any more than completely remove them. Then you'd have no cabinets, because we don't have the funds to replace them with stainless steel. That would cost a hundred thousand dollars. Besides, I feel that those cabinets have outgassed a lot. The potential for them to outgas is much, much greater than with the plaster."

For Crecelius, then, the plaster walls constitute the main problem. Happily, it's a problem for which there might be a solution: seal them. "We may end up putting sealer on the units," she says. "I hope we can eventually do that. But one of our major concerns is that the sealer is going to make it worse, because it will be more toxic than the plaster. Some of these sealers are thought to be nontoxic once they cure. Whether they are or not is another question. And while they're being painted they do definitely have an odor. So another problem is that some people may not be able to come into their apartments for a long time. And we have no funds to find people safe places to live in the meanwhile."

Crecelius hopes to ease up to the problem gingerly, by doing a kind of dry run — sealing the walls in one unit and watching to see what happens. "I hope that eventually we will be able to try some sealer on walls in one location, carefully venting the area," she says. "We could do it in the community room. We'll have to create some negative pressure inside, and using long ducting, vent out a hundred feet away while we're doing the painting. And notify people well ahead of time, so they can leave the property."

But straightforward as that tack may seem, when it comes to MCS nothing is ever without complications. The very restrictions built into the bylaws of the complex stand in their way. "We had in our rules that no paints or sealers could be used," Crecelius explains. "We're now in the process of changing those rules, but with a project with HUD funding, regulations are such that you just can't up and change your rules. You have to notify tenants in writing, notify HUD in writing. We're going through that process now. So far we haven't been able to get any consensus among the tenants that this is a good thing to do."

She shrugs. "When it gets right down to it, once we get the rules changed and move ahead to do this, it wouldn't surprise me if nobody wants to participate."

Meanwhile, life — such as it is — goes on at Ecology House. What began as such a hopeful project is now characterized by strain — strain between the residents and the physical structure, strain among the residents themselves, strain between the residents and the board members.

"I don't scream at the residents, they don't scream at me," says Crecelius. "But every single property management issue that you'd normally come up against is different, tougher, more complicated in this case."

"I can't hate the board," says Molloy. "They knocked themselves out for five years trying to make this thing happen. They spilled their guts trying to make this work, for no money. And they get kicked in the teeth for it by people who are legitimately, unbearably ill. And really resentful.

"I watched Katie for several years working her guts out for free on this thing because she just plain believed in it. Now she's mad, and feeling unappreciated — which she is. And she's not very flexible at this point about stuff. She's a much maligned person. I love her to pieces. I think she screwed up, but I had the privilege of watching her in action working her heart out for years.

"I wish we would've had some kind of collective thought like, 'Okay, given that this place is a compromise at best, we don't dare let extremely sensitive people move in here during the first year or longer till we work the bugs out. We need a bunch of normal people to live here, or people with other disabilities that don't include a dinged-up immune system. Because we're going to have to keep making repairs, and working on this place, sealing it, messing with cupboards and all sorts of stuff during the first year, the people we *don't* want in here are the most sensitive people.'

"If we could have done that, I would have a clear conscience that we had admitted defeat, let other people move in, and started repairs with well people there. Then moved them out. It would have been awful. I don't know how we could have done that. But at least we wouldn't have inflicted more chemical nightmare on these people.

"I don't think we did anybody a favor letting them move in this first year. I think we bear a lot of responsibility for what happened to those guys. I'm glad the place got built, because it is slightly better than the alternative, but I'll never be proud of it."

In the end, however, it may be that Ecology House was jinxed from the beginning. The very premise — building a safe dwelling for eleven diverse, randomly selected chemically sensitive people — may simply be unrealistic. The disease is too variable, people who suffer it too disparate, remedies too amorphous. As Katie Crecelius says, "You really can't engineer a bubble."

Chapter **2**

Bad Seeds

IF MULTIPLE CHEMICAL sensitivity is real, if it is a discrete, recognizable disease, a question arises — for physicians a very important question. "Allergic to the Twentieth Century," to the contrary, does MCS really and truly have anything to do with allergies?

At first glance you might think so. "Heightened sensitivity to a substance that in similar amounts is harmless to the majority of the group" — that's the way *Funk & Wagnalls* defines "allergy," and it's a pretty good description of MCS as well. But to let the question go at that is too easy. For when you enter the domain of allergy, and allergists, you enter a world that is rigidly prescribed and zealously guarded. The reason may be that allergy as a field, and allergists as a profession, are Johnnies-come-lately to the medical craft. And allergy, the illness they struggle to understand, is devious and strange. There's a lack of consensus as to the reason for the affliction. The treatments allergists come up with smack as much of black magic as of solid science. Allergists have had to fight hard for their turf — that battle goes on. New ailments, especially one as mysterious and difficult as MCS, are simply not readily accepted into the fold. But while the miseries caused by allergies are as old as recorded history, the fold — that is, the medical field of allergy — is relatively brand-new.

In 1902 Prince Alfred of Monaco set sail for the Mediterranean. With him on the royal yacht were two French physiologists, Charles Richet and Paul Portier. The prince had good reason for bringing the scientists along: vacationers were avoiding his Monte Carlo beach because of sea anemones. He wanted a treatment for their poisonous stings. There on board the scientists (the prince himself was an amateur oceanographer) began experiments. And when Richet and Portier returned to France, they continued the work. They knew that when exposed to weakened doses of a poison or infectious organism, the body builds up defenses. Such was the strategy behind the new miracle of vaccines and the recently developed cures for tetanus and diphtheria. Richet and Portier tried the same approach in an attempt to produce an antidote to sea anemone poison.

They were in for a surprise. They started by injecting a weakened dose of poison into laboratory dogs. This first exposure went as expected — nothing happened. The partners waited a few weeks and then, anticipating that further injections would begin to build up immunity, gave the dogs new doses of the diluted toxin. To their surprise and horror, the animals collapsed and died. In particular, it was the fatal reaction of one previously robust dog that convinced Richet and Portier of the truth of their findings. The pooch is now famous in allergy circles. Its name, appropriately enough for an investigation of sea creatures inspired by a sea cruise, was Neptune.

"The most typical experiment, that in which the result was indisputable, was carried out on a particularly healthy dog," Richet wrote. "It was given at first .1 c.c. of the glycerin extract without becoming ill; twenty-two days later, as it was in perfect health, I gave a second injection of the same amount. In a few seconds it was extremely ill; breathing became distressful and panting; it could scarcely drag itself along, lay on its side, was seized with diarrhea, vomited blood, and died in twenty-five minutes."

Rather than developing resistance, Neptune had suddenly become sensitive to the poison. Richet called the phenomenon anaphylaxis. "Anaphylaxis is the opposite condition to protection (phylaxis). I coined the word . . . to describe the peculiar attribute which certain poisons possess of increasing instead of diminishing the sensitivity of an organism to their action. . . . Accumulation is not the cause: for at the end of three, four, or five days there is no anaphylaxis; at least two or three weeks must elapse before it appears. These two factors — (a) increased sensitivity to a poison after previous injection of the same poison, and (b) an incubation period necessary for this state of increased sensitivity to develop — constitute the two essential and sufficient conditions for anaphylaxis."

We know now that all allergies work in just this fashion — initial exposure to an allergen and then a sudden exquisite sensitivity to the same, previously innocuous, substance. Richet and Portier's discovery led to the acceptance of sensitization as a separate type of immune disorder. From this point on, allergies became a distinct field of investigation.

How does this strange process of allergic sensitization come about? As it turns out, it's a marvel of perhaps wrongly directed aggression. Allergy involves a process unlike almost any other.

Normally, when our body is faced with hazardous invaders such as viruses or bacteria, our immune systems produce billions upon billions of Y-shaped bits of protein called antibodies. These tiny molecules act as an advance guard. They travel freely in the bloodstream until they encounter invading microbes. Then they go to work: they seize the intruders, disable them, and provide a target for the immune system's killers, white blood cells called lymphocytes. These antimicrobial antibodies are of the type known as IgG — immunoglobulin G. They are the most common antibodies of the immune system. And their deployment is called an immune reaction.

When it comes to specks of pollen or other allergens, however, a different mechanism springs into action. Again the body churns out antibodies, but not nearly so many, and this time they're of a type called IgE. Rather than intercepting the foreign particle and marking it for destruction as IgG would do, IgE acts curiously. It ignores the intruder and lodges tail-first onto the surface of special cells, the most prominent being mast cells. These cells are found wherever the body comes into contact with the outside world and therefore with allergens — in the skin; in the mucous membranes of the eyes, nose, and throat; and in the lining of the lungs and gut. Each of these unusual cells encloses large, globular granules, a thousand or more of them. Thus the term "mast" cell, from the German for "a fattening feed," because when discovered in the late nineteenth century, it was assumed that the cells had gobbled up the granules. By the time this rooting of IgE molecules is complete, each mast cell plays host to between one hundred thousand and five hundred thousand antibodies protruding from its surface like a forest of diminutive trees.

Now the body is primed and ready. Should other pollen invasions come — and allergy sufferers know they always do — a bizarre chain reaction takes place. When a grain of pollen happens to stick to the arms of at least two IgE antibodies — a likely occurrence considering how densely the little Ys poke out from the surface of the mast cell — it's as if a biochemical circuit closes. An explosive series of events is set into motion that ends with the mast cell bursting open and spewing forth its bellyful of granules.

The granules, in turn, contain a pharmacopeia of histamines and other chemicals, at least twenty-eight of them, that infiltrate the skin and other tissues close to the activated mast cells. These chemicals cause all the symptoms of inflammation — swelling, itching, excess mucus secretion, dilated and leaky blood vessels. The result is the familiar torture of hay fever — sniffing, sneezing, coughing, tearing. If the invaders happen to be dust mites that make their way to the lungs, the allergic reaction can generate the wheezing and shortness of breath associated with asthma. A meal of shellfish can trigger the upset stomach and diarrhea of food allergy. Peanuts or insect stings can provoke such an overwhelming explosion of these symptoms — anaphylactic shock — that the result can be death within seconds. All because of a seemingly needless reaction to harmless specks of foreign protein.

At the moment, to the misery of millions, there's no reliable method to quell the allergic reaction. Antihistamines and decongestants work for some people, some of the time, but often cause unwelcome side effects such as drowsiness. Allergy shots are not dependable — they're effective no more than half the time. They're based on the hope that when allergens are injected directly into the bloodstream, the body will loose IgG antibodies against them — in other words, mount an *immune* reaction — blocking the allergens before IgE can instigate an allergic response. Sometimes the ploy works, and with repeated injections over years allergy sufferers find themselves less likely to respond to allergens in the environment. But sometimes it doesn't. In that case, people can experience allergic reactions right there in the allergist's office. In fact, after receiving allergy shots people commonly wait in the office fifteen to twenty minutes to make sure they don't have an anaphylactic reaction.

Why does the body indulge itself in such disastrous fireworks? No one knows. But there are some intriguing theories. And none more so than that espoused by Eric Ottesen.

* * *

Ottesen is a World Health Organization allergy and parasite specialist who used to do his research at the National Institute of Allergy and Infectious Disease outside Washington, D.C. Surprisingly — or not so, considering his specialties — Ottesen suspects that allergies and parasites are linked. That is, there is an inverse relationship between allergies and the presence of parasitic worms. Find worms, you won't find allergies. Lots of allergies, few worms.

Ottesen isn't the first to suspect such a connection — which has come to be called the helminth hypothesis (from the Greek "helminth," meaning worm). But with his dual expertise in parasitology and allergy, he may be the most qualified to do so. And it's not as odd an idea as it first seems. As noted, allergies involve an unusual immune system mechanism, the IgE response. You'd have to look long and hard to find another occasion when the body employs IgE rather than its arsenal of other antibodies. But parasitic worms provoke the same IgE response. Could allergies result when the body's mechanism for getting rid of worms somehow becomes misdirected? "There must be a reason for having the allergic mechanism," Ottesen says. "It probably evolved first to fight parasite infections, and at least forty percent of the world's population is infected by parasitic worms. But when there are no parasites around, you're left with this honed immune system looking for something to attack. And those people who would have been protected in the jungle are now stuck in New York or someplace where parasites are scarce, wheezing and coughing because of pollen blowing down the street. Parasites and allergies — it's an absolutely critical relationship."

It's an intriguing theory. It isn't like nature to waste so much energy. That the allergic response may have originated as an antiparasite defense gives it a purpose. Take, for example, filarial worms and hookworms, which enter the body directly through the skin. An immune response that causes the area to become inflamed and swollen may wall off the worms and prevent them from burrowing farther. What's more, when IgE provokes mast cells into action they attract an unusual roving white blood cell called an eosinophil, which itself contains granules. The eosinophil also goes after the parasite. "It dumps its granules onto the surface of the worm," says Ottesen. "The granules contain chemicals that burn holes in the parasite until it falls to pieces." Small wonder, then, that Ottesen says, "You want to have an inflammatory response to parasites to protect yourself from penetration."

Intestinal worms such as pinworms, on the other hand, enter through the mouth — often traveling in food or water contaminated with fecal matter — then make their way to the gut. Diarrhea and vomiting, which result when the inflamed gut pours out fluid and mucus, might flush them out before they can infiltrate the intestinal wall. A number of these worms, including those that cause the widespread tropical disease schistosomiasis (sometimes called snail fever because the schistosome worm is spread by water snails), also spend part of their elaborate life cycle in the human lung. The coughing and sneezing triggered by inflammation in the airways might be the immune system's attempt to dislodge worms that have found their way into the respiratory tract. These inflammatory responses tend to be more pronounced in newcomers to the parasite-filled tropics than in those who have encountered the worms before. And they are by no means foolproof — some worms still manage to make themselves at home in the human body, establishing a chronic infection. But on the whole, the IgE response seems to do a fine job of keeping the world of worms at bay.

The point is, the seemingly unnecessary allergic mechanism and the useful parasite defense are almost identical. The theory of evolution suggests that nature retains those processes that are useful for survival and jettisons those that aren't. Therefore, useless allergies may be no more than a misapplication of the useful mechanism of parasite defense. That's why the body keeps it around. "There's got to be selective pressure for the allergic mechanism," says Ottesen. "It's so common that it's bound to be doing something useful. The only way it ever would've gotten here is because it's better to have it than not." Better, that is, because its real purpose is to attack wormy parasites. *That* is what it's there for.

If so, it should follow that the more parasitic worms in the environment, the fewer allergies people would suffer, as it's unlikely that this unique arm of the immune system could go after pollen and dust mites when its IgE antibodies are busy fighting off worms. And vice versa: the fewer parasites to contend with, the more likely that unemployed IgE would target pollen and other allergens instead.

Ottesen himself has found just such evidence in the South Pacific island of Mauke, which he last visited in 1992. What he and his cohorts discovered was that compared to their first visit twenty-one years earlier, there was much less filarial worm infection on Mauke. Only 16 percent of the population harbored the microscopic worms, as opposed to 35 percent on his first visit. The reduction resulted primarily from treating the islanders with the antiparasite drug diethylcarbamazine, which Ottesen had initiated during his earlier visit. But what Ottesen didn't bargain on was the increase in allergies. "There's no question that there was a heck of a lot more allergy out there this last time. Twenty-one years ago barely three percent of the people had allergies. This time it was at least fifteen percent." The complaints ranged from eczema to hay fever to asthma, with the most frequent affliction being food allergies.

Perhaps, suspects Ottesen, this increase in allergies is a consequence of the lack of worm infection. Perhaps the IgE defense mechanism, no longer occupied with attacking worms, is now going after new targets.

The trouble is, it's awfully hard to prove the notion one way or the other. The scope and effectiveness of our immune defenses are genetically determined; they vary from person to person. Allergies are a prime example. While one person may mount a debilitating IgE response to peanuts, say, another may react mildly, and another not at all. The same goes for parasites — not everyone reacts to the same worms with equal intensity. That makes it tough to pin down the exact nature of the relationship between parasites and allergies. "It's extraordinarily difficult to design an experiment that would confirm the inverse relationship," says Ottesen. "There are too many variables. No two people have precisely the same immune responses, and no two people have the same exposure to allergens or parasites. It's just not an easy question to answer." And it's not simply a matter of curing a few people of their parasites and then seeing if they develop allergies. To get anything approaching meaningful results, you'd have to follow large populations over long periods of time, or somehow simulate the human situation in animals.

Nevertheless, researchers are trying. For example, experiments show that rats infected by worms have weak allergic reactions, as though their battle with parasites leaves the IgE response with little ammunition for allergens. In humans, studies of immigrants from the Philippines, China, and the West Indies, where parasite infestation is high, reveal that these people have virtually no allergies — while their parasite-free offspring born in the United States and England are miserable with them.

But not all studies point in the same direction. In rural New Guinea, for example, parasite infection seems to have no effect on the prevalence of at least one allergic condition, asthma. Nor is it easy to explain why the immune system, no matter how badly underemployed and misdirected, should target invaders as inoffensive as dust mites and pollen. "It may be that allergens, like parasites, present some characteristic molecular component or shape that induces an IgE response," says Otte-sen. "But nobody has a handle on that yet."

Margie Profet thinks she does. And she doesn't think much of Ottesen's proposed allergy-parasite connection. "I more than doubt it," she says. "It would be ludicrous if allergies were here because of parasites. Natural selection just doesn't come up with such a faulty design." Rather, she proposes that far from being a useless, accidental affliction, allergies serve an impor-tant purpose. In her view, the allergic response is actually a last line of defense against toxins. Thus the explosive nature of the allergic reaction. All that swelling, sneezing, coughing, diar-rhea, and vomiting serve quickly to block or flush toxins from the system.

It's an unconventional point of view. But Profet is busy making a pretty good career out of espousing unconventional points of view. A thirty-eight-year-old theoretical biologist (the label that probably closest describes what she does), Profet is affiliated with no institution, teaches no classes, gives no lec-tures. She doesn't even hold a degree in biology (her degrees are in political philosophy, from Harvard, and physics, from the University of California at Berkeley). Nevertheless, her writing on allergies, and another paper arguing that menstruation acts as a defense against pathogens transported by sperm, have won her national attention, not to mention a $250,000 MacArthur Foundation "genius" award.

Profet's allergy-toxin hypothesis goes like this: The aller-gic response — that is, the IgE response — is unlike other immune-system process in that it utilizes nonimmunological mechanisms. Rather than gobbling up or destroying invading microorganisms, which is pretty much what the "normal" im-mune response is all about, the allergic response attempts to expel the invaders. All that sneezing, tearing, vomiting, diar-rhea — those are nonimmunological strategies for getting rid of the intruders, fast. "Fast" is the key. The allergic response can be immediate. Enter the intruder — *boom!* It's catapulted out. This is a powerful response, in Profet's term an "evolved" response. It just didn't make sense to her that something so sophisticated might be the accidental offshoot of something else.

What, then, has the allergic response evolved to expel? Toxins. Toxins are just about everywhere. Plants produce toxins as a defense against being infected by microorganisms and eaten by animals and insects. Insects, reptiles, and marine animals produce toxins as a defense against predators or to disable prey. Bacteria produce toxins. And certain naturally occurring metals, such as nickel and lead, are toxic. We encounter toxins all the time.

What does all that have to do with allergies? Profet contends that common allergens contain a variety of toxins. For example, pollen grains may contain phenolic acids and alkaloids, and hay dust is often infested by toxic fungal spores. And even if an allergen may not itself be toxic, it may be a carrier for toxins and thus provoke the allergic defense. Seemingly innocuous allergens like animal dander, for example, can transport piggy-backing toxins encountered during the animal's meanderings. And once the body associates the allergen with its hitchhiking toxin, the allergen itself becomes the target.

But allergies aren't our first line of defense against toxins. "When you're around toxins for some time, you build up detoxification enzymes against those particular toxins," Profet explains. Skin and mucous secretions keep them away, as does our constant sluffing of skin and the surface of our respiratory system and gut, those areas that have contact with the outside world. Enzymes and antibodies in the linings of the respiratory and digestive systems break down toxins. And powerful enzymes in the liver and kidneys destroy anything that slips through. It's when these primary defenses don't work, or when people are exposed to new toxins — when moving to a new town, for example — that allergies spring to the rescue.

"Allergies are a last line of defense. They're a very risky thing," Profet says. That much is certainly true. The allergic reaction can be so quick and powerful that the ostensibly protective response to that toxin-carrying peanut can cause death. Or, like a smoke detector that sounds a false alarm, the allergic response may go after a truly innocuous invader. It's the price we pay for protection. Allergies may be well evolved, but they're not perfect.

For Profet, then, the notion that the allergic response is an unfortunate byproduct of a defense against parasitic worms is simply ludicrous. If anything, the truth is just the other way around. "If allergy had evolved primarily to protect against helminths, it would represent astonishing poor design by natural selection," she writes. "However, it is possible that some of the mechanisms of allergy have been co-opted or altered for defense against helminths."

Therefore, having allergies, or at least the capability to have them, is worthwhile rather than bothersome. "Somebody with the full capacity for allergies who has none is probably very healthy," Profet says. "It means their detoxification enzymes are detoxifying everything. But if they don't have a capacity for allergies, or if they have a low capacity, then they may be in trouble. They're more likely to get harmed, irreparably harmed, if they're exposed to toxins repeatedly. The allergic adaptation is there for a reason."

In fact, contends Profet, allergies may even help prevent cancer. Those expelled toxins may include carcinogens and other cancer-causing substances. She cites studies measuring the correlation between allergies and cancer. In almost three-quarters of these studies, people with allergies were less likely to develop cancer. By way of explanation, Profet points out that most human cancers arise in the lining of the gut, the skin, the lungs, those very surfaces that come into contact with the outside environment and its plethora of toxins and carcinogens. It's these surfaces that are lined by mast cells and IgE antibodies. In other words, the allergic response occurs precisely where it's most needed.

Eric Ottesen is unimpressed. "The notion sounds somewhat contrived. It's making something fit a theory rather than the facts begging you to create the theory. But," he says with a shrug, "until somebody proves the point, one hypothesis is as good as another."

Meanwhile, worms or no worms, toxins or no toxins, defensive strategy or useless misery, allergies endure.

Is MCS one of these allergies? Hardcore allergists say no. The hallmark of allergy is an IgE reaction, and people with MCS don't necessarily display elevated levels of IgE. Therefore MCS is not an allergy. In fact, the lack of a generally accepted, reliable marker is one of the mysteries surrounding the affliction.

Another involves the nature of the miseries experienced by MCS sufferers. While sometimes these symptoms resemble those of allergies, sometimes they seem alien. For example, the worst of Rick Kiessig's afflictions — profound fatigue and the inability to think, what he calls "brain fog" — are not your typical allergic symptoms. Although a hay fever sufferer, say, wiped out and miserable from sneezing and sniffing, might experience similar problems, the severity and persistence of the symptoms associated with MCS are decidedly un–allergy-like. As are the paralysis and numbness Kiessig endures, the memory lapses that plague some, the heart problems others have experienced, the problems with balance, coordination, and sensation experienced by still others. These are complaints more suitable for a neurologist, cardiologist, internist, or psychiatrist than allergist.

But why? Why should the "heightened sensitivity" of allergy be limited to a certain kind of immune reaction producing certain kinds of problems? In the early days the field wasn't so restricted. In 1906 when a Viennese pediatrician named

Clemens von Pirquet coined the term "allergy" (from the Greek for "other" and "work"), he used it to "designate this general concept of *altered capacity to react.*" Then the mere fact of heightened sensitivity and altered reactivity was the key.

But as the new field flourished and allergists strove for respectability, they began to adopt a more narrow definition of their craft — a more "scientific" definition. It's easy to forget in these days of celebrity viruses and drug-resistant bacteria that at the turn of the century the notion of disease being caused by agents outside the body, much less invisible "germs," was brand-new and quite unsettling. It had been thought for centuries that disease was a manifestation of bodily imbalance. In the late nineteenth century, Louis Pasteur in France and Robert Koch in Germany exploded that concept by dramatically demonstrating that microbes can cause disease. Pasteur singlehandedly saved France's silk industry by showing how to control the microbe that was killing the country's silkworms. He also developed a vaccine against rabies. Koch identified the microbe that caused anthrax, a fatal disease of animals as well as of humans, and tracked down the tuberculosis bacterium. And, following their lead, the Englishman Joseph Lister (whose name is memorialized in the mouthwash Listerine) popularized sterile surgery, saving uncountable lives.

This "germ theory" of disease made its way across the Atlantic, and, with Johns Hopkins in the lead, by the turn of the century American medical institutions were teaching the new gospel. No wonder that in the 1920s, as people were discovering the microbe-fighting mechanisms of the immune system, the fledgling field of allergy fell in line. In response to the urging of European allergists, an allergy became defined as "the consequence of an immune reaction." The proof was that when blood was transferred from an allergy sufferer to a "normal" person, that person started having allergic reactions. There must be some immune agent in allergy blood, therefore, that mediated the condition. No one knew what the agent was, but it was given the name "Reagin." As a result of this new direction, gone was the original notion of a general hypersensitivity to a wide variety of annoyances.

It wasn't until many years later, however, that allergists pinned down their immune agent. In 1967 a Japanese husband-and-wife research team working at Yale Medical School, Kimishige and Teruko Ishizaka, discovered that Reagin was in fact IgE. Soon after that they described how IgE combines with mast cells to release histamine and other chemicals that cause the allergic reaction. All of us have IgE in our immune system armamentarium — allergy sufferers simply have abnormally large amounts. Still, however, some things don't quite add up. For example, certain people with asthma do not display unusually high levels of IgE, yet they continue to suffer. Why? No one knows. In fact, only a relatively small percentage of allergy sufferers display elevated levels of IgE in their blood. What is going on with the rest of them? And when it comes to allergy shots, it turns out that even when they relieve allergies, the IgE levels in patients' blood doesn't necessarily drop. In some cases it remains elevated for a year or more. Why? No one knows. Mysteries remain.

Nevertheless, most allergists have been loath to accept MCS into the field. The upshot has been that the symptoms of MCS, and the people who suffer them, have fallen through the cracks. Faced with infirmities that don't fit into their canon, many allergists simply dismiss MCS sufferers, all too often suggesting that their real problem is not in their lungs, or their skin, or their stomach, or their joints, or the myriad other places where MCS symptoms manifest themselves, but in their heads. That is, these people should be seeing a psychiatrist rather than an allergist.

Given that vacuum, it's not surprising that like flowers pushing through cracks in a sidewalk (or weeds, depending on your point of view), a new kind of allergist has sprung into being. These docs call themselves clinical ecologists, or environ-

mental physicians, and they emphasize the role of the environment in disease. While generally discredited by conventional
allergists and other physicians, they've provided a sympathetic
ear for MCS sufferers, a conviction that MCS is indeed a valid
problem, and an approach toward treating the disorder. The
pioneer of this new breed was Theron Randolph.

Chapter **3**

Emptying the Barrel

THERON RANDOLPH DIED on September 29, 1995. He was eighty-nine years old. In his obituary, his hometown *Chicago Tribune* called him "the most exceptional and outstanding physician in the entire field of allergy." The *New York Times* said that "traditional medical bodies like the American College of Allergy and Immunology, which contended there was no scientific basis for his approach, are sharply skeptical of Dr. Randolph's unorthodox therapies."

The disagreement is typical. It was Randolph who first fully recognized the problem of multiple chemical sensitivity, Randolph who developed a controversial brand of medicine, which he dubbed clinical ecology, to deal with the disorder, Randolph who cofounded the Society for Clinical Ecology (now called the American Academy of Environmental Medicine, or AAEM), Randolph who more than anyone inspired other physicians to head in this direction, patients to enter their offices, and conventional practitioners to blow their tops. No wonder he's praised and reviled — it all depends on your point of view.

Talk to his patients, however, and many of them express the same point of view: Randolph helped them. The first MCS patient he helped — at least the one who convinced him that there was such a thing as chemical sensitivity — was a former cosmetics saleswoman and doctor's wife named Nora Barnes. It was 1947, and Randolph was a board-certified allergist on the faculty of Northwestern University Medical School in Chicago. Barnes came to his office complaining of a bewildering variety of problems: bronchial asthma, persistent fatigue, irritability, depression, fluctuations in weight, headaches that sent her hurrying to bed, even intermittent loss of consciousness. No one could find a cause for her problems. Her doctors had diagnosed her as a hypochondriac.

Randolph, however, detected clues to the cause of her condition — but none of them, in combination with the others, suggested any pattern. Applying nail polish made Barnes's eyes itch — she used makeup to hide the redness and inflammation. Driving into Chicago from her home state of Michigan made her sick. On three occasions she collapsed while driving. She often became ill when riding in the backseat of automobiles but more rarely in the front. Autos with noisy mufflers were especially hard on her. And, Randolph remembered in his memoirs, "Arriving at a hotel in Chicago's downtown Loop district, she was practically incoherent when she called me on the telephone. By chance, the desk clerk gave her a room on the twenty-third floor. Soon she felt somewhat better and attempted to go downstairs and do some shopping. But she found that when she went into the lobby or onto any floor below the twentieth, her nausea, dizziness, and feelings of suffocation returned." And perhaps the most puzzling clue of all was the fact that Barnes became miserable and "neurotic" every Fourth of July and didn't improve until summer was over. An obvious possibility was hay fever, but people rarely suffered hay fever in the summer in that part of the country.

Randolph was stumped. But he was determined to get to the bottom of Barnes's problems. "He did two things that were really intelligent," remembers Denver environmental physician Kendall Gerdes, who trained with Randolph. "One was to see the lady for free. So if he spent a lot of time with her, it was simply time invested — he wasn't taking money out of her pocket. Secondly, he decided that he would presume there was an answer out there, and he was simply going to wait until it appeared."

He waited four years. By that time he had accumulated fifty pages of single-spaced typewritten notes concerning Barnes's case, gleaned, as was his habit with his patients, from asking her an enormous number of questions and, without reaction, recording her answers on his manual typewriter. "This routine proved to be so helpful in dealing with alleged hypochondriacs that I adopted the technique of practicing 'poker faced medicine,'" Randolph wrote. By not reacting one way or another he encouraged patients to report their conditions honestly and accurately, providing him "data independent of snap judgments."

One April day in 1951 a fierce storm lambasted the Chicago area. All Randolph's other patients canceled their appointments. Only Barnes, already in town from Michigan, came to the office. Now, with plenty of time to spare, Randolph sat her down and together they read through his fifty pages of notes. "By the time I had finished rereading one-third of the history and progress notes I realized that there was, indeed, a common denominator extending through this report," he remembered. "Almost all her problems could be traced back to petrochemicals, combustion products, or man-made chemicals manufactured from petroleum. Nora Barnes was allergic or susceptible to a wide range of supposedly safe environmental agents."

Today an environmental doc would suspect such a connection immediately. In 1951, however, Randolph was breaking new ground. With this realization, suddenly everything made sense. Why did the odor of her gas range and other gas appliances make Barnes sick? Because of combustion. Why did she react to plastic-encased furniture and sponge-rubber padding? Because they were petroleum-derived products. Why did her health fall apart while driving to Randolph's office? Because she had to pass through northern Indiana's industrial belt and its proliferation of petroleum- and combustion products. And why did she do better in the upper floors of Chicago hotels? Because up there she was removed from the city's street-level pollution. "She had learned to stay on the top floor of the tallest hotel in Chicago where she recovered more rapidly than elsewhere," Randolph remembered. "But even so, one and one-half to two days were necessary before she improved sufficiently to be able to come to my office. A few times between 1948 and 1950 I saw her on the twenty-sixth floor of her hotel when it was still possible to look down on the ceiling of air pollution existing in Chicago."

Little by little Randolph began to decipher other mysteries about Barnes's condition. For example, canned tomatoes made her ill, but tomatoes from her own garden or tomatoes stored in glass containers did not. Randolph traced the problem to the lining of the cans (which contained resins of phenol, a chemical used in disinfectants). Maraschino cherries, mint sauce, and hot dogs agitated her, and drinking crème de menthe made her so sick she passed out. Randolph determined that she was sensitive to food colorings. And what about her strange Fourth of July miseries? It turned out that Barnes and her husband had a cabin in the woods where they spent their summers — from July 4th on! Barnes was allergic to pine. She couldn't tolerate the cabin's pine paneling, burning pine in the fireplace, or various other pine-scented materials, including disinfectants. When Barnes removed these products from the cabin, she felt better.

Soon enough it became obvious to Randolph that he was on to something important. "The case of Nora Barnes provided a new perspective on medical practice," he wrote. "It soon became apparent that she was not alone, that other patients seen by physicians with similarly peculiar and multiple symptoms were actually suffering from allergies to synthetic chemicals. These people were not born this way. They acquired a high susceptibility because of constant day-in and day-out exposure to chemicals, especially in the period since World War Two."

Moreover, these unconventional allergies involved unconventional symptoms — neurological symptoms, psychological symptoms — such as depression, confusion, fatigue, irritability, loss of coordination. But like conventional allergies, allergies to chemicals could be at least partially alleviated by avoiding the irritant.

It was a watershed case for Randolph, the beginning of the wider recognition that an affliction as bizarre and puzzling as multiple chemical sensitivity might be real. "Until the end of his life Randolph kept Barnes's chart around," says Gerdes. "It was a testament to his ability to defer judgment until he found an answer."

Ironically, however, the very method by which he had deciphered Barnes's problem — deduction from extensive observation — later provoked the criticism that continues to haunt environmental medicine: that it is unscientific and unsubstantiated. Randolph had not arrived at his diagnosis by finding a blood marker like IgE, for example. Nor had he found any other consistent physiological signs. No matter that observation and deduction based on experience was a time-honored method of practicing medicine — it simply wasn't scientific. And not only that, his diagnosis of chemical allergy flew in the face of the conventional wisdom in the field. It's no wonder that environmental medicine, and its headline ailment, multiple chemical sensitivity, have been thrown out of the halls of orthodox medicine.

Randolph never forgot or forgave. "The allergists are stuck in a trap of their own making," he said. "There are numerous mechanisms in allergy. It's ridiculous to limit the concept of hypersensitivity to the one mechanism of IgE. They're trying to make it an exclusive practice. They won't give up. Why? Because they're blockheads."

Nor did he deviate from the lonely direction he had established. And today it's no longer lonely. Randolph's influence has been enormous. In 1987 Randolph estimated that environmental medicine practitioners numbered nearly two thousand, as opposed to three thousand to thirty-five hundred conventional allergists. ("When there were only a few of us we were treated as gadflies. Now that we are forty percent of the total we are perceived as a real threat and dealt with accordingly.") The American Academy of Environmental Medicine, the organization Randolph cofounded in 1965, estimates a similar number. The organization now numbers six hundred dues-paying members and considers them to represent a third to a quarter of the total of practicing environmental physicians. The AAEM's yearly meeting is a multiday marathon of talks, exhibits, sightseeing, and socializing. Among the events in the fall 1995 gathering in Tucson, Arizona, was an unscheduled presentation: a memorial to Theron Randolph.

Although in the latter part of his long career Randolph ran his own clinic, complete with nurses, visiting physicians, and interns, the image persists of the lone, pioneering doc banging the keys of his typewriter while distressed patients pour out their life stories. It's quite a jump to Bill Rea and his Environmental Health Center in Dallas.

Enter this world, and you're in a sophisticated, high-tech treatment facility. The Environmental Health Center (or EHC-Dallas) staff includes Rea and two other physicians, Alfred Johnson and Gerald Ross, nutritionists, counselors, physical therapists, nurses and technicians, an on-site lab, and working relationships with two psychiatrists and two psychologists — seventy-five people in all. The waiting room looks like something out of *Star Wars:* transparent glass entry and door, glass-covered walls, shiny marble tile floors, high white ceiling covered by nontoxic paint. A TV recessed behind glass continuously screens a scary film about the evils of pesticide use throughout the world. Clean air flows in through a filtered circulation system. White-coated staff sequestered behind small sliding glass windows tend to a constant stream of patients — some wearing respirators, some in wheelchairs — who await their turn in hardwood chairs. Many of them have come to the center in desperation, having already gone through the futility of seeing conventional physicians. They are some of the sickest people in the world.

There are none of the comforts of your typical doctor's office here. The effect is at once reassuring (this is a clean, uncontaminated, safe place) and cold (what in hell am I getting into?).

A sign outside the office offers guidelines:

No Aftershave. No Perfume.

No Cologne. Pesticide-Free.

Across a narrow, gloomy hall a small shop offers environmentally safe products. Here you can buy books and pamphlets about MCS (including three thick volumes authored by Rea), air filters and undyed cotton clothing, vitamins and herbal supplements, organic snacks. Meanwhile, people scurry along the hall, disappearing behind doors. This place is *busy*, like some underground hive completely separated from the outside world.

And presiding over all of it is Bill Rea. I was forewarned that Rea is a strong personality, a "cowboy." He's busy, brash, hard to pin down. If he trusts you, he might talk. If not, good luck. After a handful of short phone conversations, I wrote Rea asking if I might visit him, hang out at the clinic, meet some of his patients. He sent back a two-sentence reply: "You may visit the clinic. You'll have to arrange to talk to patients on your own."

Rea is sixty-one years old, sandy-haired, slim and compact, except for an ample gut accentuated by his predilection for wearing short neckties that end mid-torso, like an arrow pointing the way to his belly. He looks weathered, tired, and walks with a pronounced limp, the residue of a bout with polio when he was six months old. "I started off with a little handicap," he says with an ironic grin. "Helped me decide to go into medicine. Taught me you have to believe what you see, not what you hear."

Like Randolph, who grew up on a farm in Michigan, Rea is a midwestern farm boy, from Ohio. He still sounds like a farm boy — blunt, plainspoken, often ending his sentences with an abrupt "okay?" to drive home the point. "About thirty years ago I was working on the linings for artificial lungs and hearts, okay?" he says. (Rea is unique among MCS docs in that he was a surgeon — a cardiovascular surgeon — before he became an environmental doc. He still thinks of himself as a surgeon first, and a big chunk of his day is often spent in the operating room.) "They're still a bugaboo today. Artificial lungs and hearts have problems because they cause blood clots. When the synthetics hit the body, there's clotting. I started thinking, 'Food seems to be getting worse, air seems to be getting worse. If a synthetic hurts 'em when it's placed in there, what if they eat it or drink it or breathe it?'" He laughs. "Hey, why wouldn't it do the same thing?

"I knew about phlebitis — blood clots and inflammation of the veins. It can kill you. At that time they used to send all the people with blood clots to cardiovascular surgeons, so I had a bunch of people who were incapacitated with chronic phlebitis. I started experimenting with some of those patients and found that you could trigger clotting and all sorts of things with chemicals like phenol and formaldehyde. That's when I started putting two and two together.

"So I started working on it. I started a nonprofit foundation, raised some money, started doing research on all the materials people live with. Back then the idea of sensitivity to the environment was pretty far out — except we had seen it in lung patients. The lung is open to the outside, and every surgeon knows that environmental pollutants affect the lungs. Every surgeon knows about asbestos causing cancer of the lungs, cigarette smoke causing cancer of the lungs. You'd see black lung disease, valley fever, on and on. So the idea of sensitivity to the environment wasn't foreign to us, even though it was foreign to everybody else. To us it was common sense.

"But I wondered about that after I wrote my first paper about chemicals causing blood clotting. I sent it to the *Journal of the American Medical Association.* They said, 'This is a novel concept. Nobody on the reviewing panel has ever heard of such a thing. Therefore, we're gonna reject it.'" Rea shakes his head. "What a state American medicine is in."

"Sounds like it was an advantage coming from surgery," I say.

Rea nods vigorously. "It was a real advantage. I had no biases. In fact, I was stunned by the biases out there when I got to know Dr. Randolph and his opposition. I read his book and thought, 'This guy's got it! He understands what's going on.' I told him my experiences, and we got to be really good friends."

One of those experiences involved Rea's own sensitivity, which he first discovered in the operating room. "I found out I was sensitive to anesthetics. Then to beef, wheat, a ton of things. I would get dizzy, get problems in the inner ear." In fact, his problems were more widespread than that. Rea suffered muscle aches, joint swelling, a spastic colon, and fatigue. He couldn't tolerate odors from the laboratory, and when he inserted bronchoscopes into anesthetized patients, he developed an irregular heartbeat. His skin developed a yellow hue, and he bruised easily. He was found to be sensitive to chlorine, alcohol, formaldehyde, pesticides, and phenol.

"But I'm pretty well clear now," Rea says.

"Through your own treatment?"

"Well, yeah." He grins. "It works. How about that?"

The fact that it works has made the Environmental Health Center a mecca for chemically sensitive people all over the world. Rea and his colleagues have studied and treated over thirty thousand MCS patients. Rick and Lynn Kiessig travel to Dallas from the San Francisco Bay Area, with their son William, in tow. Annabelle Brausieck makes the five-hour trip from Wimberley; so does Sue Pitman. In fact, the presence of the clinic is one of the reasons chemically sensitive people settle in the area in the first place.

Rea's methods of treating MCS are a synthesis of already existing approaches and the clinic's own insights. They can be intricate and various, but basically the EHC-Dallas system boils down to four major emphases.

1. Avoid exposure to those things that bother you. ("Avoidance, avoidance, avoidance," chants Rea.)
2. Nutritional therapy, boosting the body's overall health by proper eating — organic food, glass-bottled spring water — rotation diets, and vitamin and mineral supplements.
3. Immunotherapy, or provocation-neutralization therapy, as it's also called.
4. Heat therapy. ("If they're really chemically ill, put 'em in a heat chamber and sweat it out of 'em," Rea says. "It's similar to a sauna, but specially designed so it doesn't put out a lot of toxins.")

All this may sound bizarre to someone used to conventional medicine, and worse than that to orthodox docs. To the people who come to Dallas, however, reeling from their illnesses, smarting from the frustration of having dealt with mainstream physicians — some 80 percent of the center's patients have already seen between five and twenty doctors — the approach soon becomes second nature. Best of all, for many people it seems to work. But not without a lot of effort all around. Rick Kiessig's experience provides an object lesson, not only of the possibility of relief for people with MCS but of how hard-won that relief can be.

Kiessig first traveled to Dallas in January of 1994. He showed up at the clinic having already completed a twenty-page health questionnaire that had been mailed to him beforehand. By taking a verbal history, his doctor, Gerald Ross, fleshed out and expanded upon that information. Randolph's tradition of exhaustive patient histories is alive and well.

"Then he did a physical exam, which is not that much different from a physical you'd get at any doctor's office — weight, blood pressure, height," recalls Kiessig. "But he did a few additional things." As one of the hallmarks of MCS can be loss of coordination and equilibrium, those additional things include balance tests. For example, Ross asked Kiessig to balance on his toes with eyes closed. He couldn't do it.

Ross has another favorite test. He asks patients to keep their eyes open, put one foot directly in front of the other, heel to toe, then close their eyes and try to balance. Healthy individuals should be able to do that. If they can't, it's an indication that there may be a neurological problem stemming from chemical sensitivity.

After that comes the next weapon in the center's diagnostic arsenal: blood tests. "We start with the same basic things that would be reasonable in most disciplines of medicine," says Ross. "Reasonable" is a word Ross uses a lot. Tall, slim, graying — he's forty-nine years old — he projects a seriousness and attentiveness that invite trust. And as a native of Nova Scotia, he has a Canadian reserve that balances his enthusiasm. "Reasonable" fits. He's a good complement to Rea, with his more caustic style — like an earnest younger brother. And he too was compelled into environmental medicine by his own sensitivities.

"We do the basics of good medicine to begin with," he says. Those basics include measuring patients' white blood cells to assess immune function; red blood cells to look for anemia; blood sugar, cholesterol, and liver function to assess general health. Ross also measures the level of IgE in the blood. "It may be up in these patients, because they often have problems with classical allergies."

But he also orders up a battery of tests that you'd never see in a conventional doctor's office. "One of the unique things we do is look for evidence of chemical contamination in the blood," he says. Traces may signify the presence of chemical sensitivity. "And I almost routinely measure the minerals inside red blood cells. If patients are low in magnesium, that's almost always correlated with chronic fatigue. And chemically sensitive patients are frequently low in sulfur or selenium. If they are, they have trouble clearing toxins from their system. That's very well known in the basic science literature."

Ross also goes after what environmental docs — but not conventional physicians — consider one of the most common impediments to good health: candida yeast. "Sometimes we'll measure antibody levels against candida," he says. "That remains a controversial issue in medicine, the whole business of whether candida yeast may not be the innocuous little creature medicine has always taught that it is. But we feel that in some patients it causes significant problems."

Finally Ross measures patients' levels of nutrition. "The most frequent cause of immunosuppression is undernutrition," he says. "We usually think of toxic stuff, and that can really suppress immune function, no doubt about that. But the most frequent cause is the lack of the right nutrient fuels that drive the immune system." He tests for specific amino acids in blood and urine, and looks at the level of various vitamins.

In Kiessig, these tests showed ample evidence of chemical sensitivity. He displayed high levels of pesticides in his blood and was low in a number of vitamins and minerals, including the element sulfur. There was no doubt in Ross's mind that Kiessig's immune functions were impaired.

The final testing procedure — perhaps the most controversial technique of all — is skin testing. On the face of it, the term "skin testing" should make anyone who's ever been to a conventional allergist feel right at home. Skin testing is a staple of allergy diagnostic technique. But this is different — especially so because the testing itself leads immediately to the third of EHC-Dallas's methods of treatment, immunotherapy. In fact, instantly shutting down the reaction is part of the testing procedure. To explain, we'll take a detour to Buffalo, New York, and one of the foremost practitioners of the art, pediatric environmental allergist Doris Rapp.

Doris Rapp practices in a red brick building with a white gabled roof set back from a busy four-lane avenue. You can't miss it. Big white letters shout out the news:

Environmental Allergy Center
Doris Rapp, M.D.

A sign on the door reads:

Please knock.
Do not enter if you smell of tobacco, perfume,
hair spray, or fabric softener.

The waiting room sports two air purifiers — as well as a mass of squirming, restless kids and their harried parents.

Rapp greets me in her consultation room, a bright and cheery space that looks more like a living room than a doctor's office. "I don't like this doctor-behind-the-high-desk-looking-down business," she says. "I want people to feel at home. It's much less threatening." She's a robust sixty-eight-year-old with a handsome, craggy face, a forthright, authoritative manner, and ice blue eyes. The hackneyed expression "tough love" pops into my mind. She understands and she cares, but you better not mess with her.

Fact is, though, plenty of people have. For although Rapp has been a board-certified pediatric allergist since 1962 and is a clinical assistant professor of pediatrics at the State University of New York at Buffalo, the recipient of that institution's distinguished alumni award, and the author of some forty scientific articles and seven books, she's also an environmental physician. And that means controversy.

Much of the controversy revolves around skin testing and immunotherapy, which in Rapp's office, and Bill Rea's, consists of a time-consuming procedure called provocation-neutralization (P/N). Explains Rapp, "You provoke the symptoms that patients have at home, and then you eliminate them with a neutralizing dose of the same substance."

Here's how it works. In traditional testing, allergists inject underneath the skin a variety of tiny doses of allergy-causing substances, sometimes up to forty at a time. These are classical allergens — pollens, molds, dust mites, and the like — the substances that provoke the classical allergic reaction, the IgE response. If, after ten minutes or so, the area around any of the sites becomes red or swells like a mosquito bite — a condition called a wheal — it's likely that the patient is allergic to that particular substance. If nothing happens, the allergist tries different doses and different extracts. The doses start weak and grow stronger, with a tenfold increase in potency at each go round.

Once the offending substances reveal themselves, it's up to the allergist to decide how powerful treatment — allergy shots made up of doses of the very same substances — should be. If you sneeze a lot during pollen season but not in wintertime, the vaccine may contain more pollen than dust. If your miseries arise in a damp, moldy house in February, the vaccine will be heavy with dust and molds. Initially patients receive shots of these extracts three times a week. The idea is to develop tolerance to the exposures. After weeks to months of that routine, it's time for less frequent injections until the allergies disappear — *if* they disappear. The process can go on for years.

An environmental doc's provocation-neutralization skin testing doesn't differ much in concept, but in practice the two approaches diverge dramatically. For example, P/N doses include the classical allergens used by conventional doctors and much more besides — toxic as well as supposedly benign chemicals, common foods, extracts of air from offices and schools, perfumes, yeasts. Usually doses are injected under the skin, or intradermally; sometimes they're given in drops under the tongue, so-called sublingual testing. And they're given one at a time. That means in contrast to the traditional procedure, in which giving and gleaning results from scores of allergens may take only half an hour or so, P/N testing can last for what may seem like forever — three to six days is the norm. It's an ordeal for everyone.

Finally — and this is the most striking contrast between provocation-neutralization and traditional testing — the progression goes from strong dilution to weak, in increments of 1 to 5. "We always start with a relatively strong concentration, because we want to produce mild symptoms," says Rapp. "That's why it's called provocation." This "provocation" not only may generate a wheal, it can often reproduce the full range of allergic reactions on the spot. Then, through a "neutralizing" dose of the same allergen, an environmental doc can shut down those reactions within minutes. In other words, P/N can be both diagnostic test *and* therapy.

"We do it in a very systematic way," explains Rapp. "First of all, we take a very detailed history of your illness and figure out what the most likely culprits are. If you're worse during pollen season, regardless of what the symptoms are, we test the pollen that's in the air first. If you're worse after meals, we say, 'What're your favorite foods?' And we test those favorite foods. If you're worse in a particular situation, putting gas in your car, say, then we'd be more apt to try chemicals."

Within ten minutes after the injection, Rapp and her team look for symptoms. "Mild symptoms might be a change in the pulse, a change in breathing, a change in appearance, a change in the size of the wheal or injection site, a change in how you feel, how you act, how you behave. We check our kids' breathing. We look at their faces to see if they've got red ears or red cheeks or dark eye circles. And we check their writing and drawing." Writing and drawing, Rapp feels, especially for kids, who often can't explain their feelings verbally, provide a window to the allergic soul.

Once the injections cause one or more of these reactions, Rapp knows she's found the culprit. She then starts the neutralization part of the procedure by giving a new set of increasingly more *dilute* injections of the suspect substance. "We watch the symptoms gradually decrease," she says. "The one-in-twenty-five dilution might make you feel a little better. Then the one-to-a-hundred-and-twenty-five definitely better, but there's still a little bit of trouble. Then we put in a drop of the one-to-six-hundred-and-twenty-five dilution and everything's back to normal. That's the neutralization dose." It's this dose that her patients take home for long-term immunotherapy, receiving injections of the extract or placing it under their tongue for months or years if necessary. Along with avoiding the offending substance and bolstering general health with vitamins and minerals, this immunotherapy is the heart of Rapp's treatment regime. In time, if the approach works, it might be possible for patients to reincorporate that offending allergen, or food, or chemical into their lives.

Why? No one knows. "Immunologists have some theories,

but we really don't know how the process works," says Rapp. "All we know is that the body acts differently with different dilutions."

No matter how it may work, environmental docs claim that provocation-neutralization treatment, or immunotherapy, can reproduce, and nullify, the entire range of allergic symptoms experienced in MCS. Rapp has seen them all. And she has *recorded* them all. In order to alert other nontraditional physicians, educate the public, and give the lie to naysayers, she maintains an extensive videotape library of P/N sessions with her patients. Thousands of videos, a separate office just to house them. When Rapp says to me, "Watch this, it'll curl your eyelashes," she's right on.

There on the screen a slim, dark-haired nine-year-old named Scott smiles into the camera. His problem is wheat. So, without knowing what's coming (the technique is called "single-blinded testing," Rapp's normal procedure), he's given an injection of a tiny drop of wheat extract, the provocation dose, under the skin. In a few moments Scott turns into a monster. He shrieks. He screams. "I want to break your neck in half!" he bellows. "I want to kill! I hate everyone!" Then, after a neutralizing dose, he's once again placid, the accommodating kid he was in the beginning.

A shy eight-year-old named Marsha draws a picture of a contented little girl with bangs, just like her own, staring into space with wide, round eyes. Rapp explains: Marsha has been taking fluoride tablets for two years. Eight days after she took her first tablet she became sad, and a month later extremely depressed. Marsha has been seeing neurologists, psychologists, psychiatrists. She even spent time in a psychiatric hospital. "And no one tested for fluoride, because no one believed that fluoride could affect how she felt and how she behaved."

Marsha is given a drop of fluoride extract under the tongue.

Seven minutes later, the camera moves in for a close up. There the little girl sits, hugging her teddy bear, tears running down her cheeks.

"How do you feel now, Marsha?" Rapp asks.

"Sad. I'm still sad."

Now when Marsha draws a picture, the little girl on the page is crying. And she adds tears to the face in the picture she drew before.

Then comes the neutralizing dose. Soon Marsha draws a winsome kitten, manages a shy smile, and says she feels "good."

"Do you want to eat some lunch now?" asks Rapp.

A smile. "Yes."

A tall eleven-year-old named Edward calmly draws a detailed rendering of a fish. He has come to see Rapp because he is behaving badly at school. He receives an injection of an extract made from a sample of the air at his school. (Rapp makes air extracts by using something that looks like an aquarium pump to bubble air collected at the site through a test tube of saline. After eight hours, everything in the air that's water-soluble remains behind. Sterilize the solution, and you have an injectable extract.)

Now, after the school-air injection, making a fish or any other kind of drawing is out of the question for Edward. He throws pencils, scribbles on the wall. He crawls under the table, climbs onto the counter, marches over the couch, his mother in hot pursuit. He slaps at her, pinches her arm. "Fuck off!" he shouts to the camera.

Afterward, after a neutralizing dose, Edward calmly draws a picture of another fish, a "swordtail."

And there's an overweight eleven-year-old named Ned. Of all the videos she shows me, his is the most dramatic. He suffers from severe MCS. Rapp tests his reaction to tomatoes. Fifteen minutes afterward Ned becomes so violent he has to be held down. He spits at his mother and a doctor helping to restrain him. He shrieks that he's going insane. "I can't help it!" he cries.

"This is what he would do at school," says his mother, while struggling to pin her son's legs to the sofa. "And the principal would sit on him. He'd come home with cut lips and a bruised face. They'd lock him in a closet, tie him to a chair. They said it was a discipline problem. That his mother and father don't know how to deal with children."

As Rapp's nurses experiment to find the right neutralizing dose, Ned's violent behavior continues. He slaps at his mother, yanks the doctor's tie, laughs hysterically and screams that he "wants to kill." Finally he becomes so agitated that he tears off his clothes. There he stands — totally naked, panting, shivering, miserable.

When the nurses finally find the neutralizing dose the transformation is astonishing. Now, pants on but still shirtless, Ned sits quietly on the couch, drawing. "How are you feeling now?" he's asked.

"Much better."

"I did want to die," Ned says later. "I didn't know what was wrong with me. But now that I know I'm going to get fixed, I want to live and have a life."

I'm not the only one who finds Ned's story striking. So does Phil Donahue. After being treated for a few months, Ned and his mother appeared on the *Donahue* show, along with Rapp and a handful of her patients. Slimmed down and calmed down, smiling in a shirt and tie, Ned tells Donahue that he's glad to be there, but that it's tough because of all the perfumes and odors in the studio.

Donahue says, "You get a whiff of some kind of perfume and — "

"Whoa, I'm gone," answers Ned.

His mother then goes through the litany of Ned's life. He was misdiagnosed with Tourette's syndrome. He was allergic to just about everything except pork and soy. Milk caused chronic bed-wetting. Natural gas caused severe tics. Electromagnetic waves from TV sets and computers and microwaves made Ned violent. And there sits Ned taking it all in, twitching a little, a little ill at ease, but composed and quiet, with a clear, friendly gaze.

"We got a hundred and forty thousand letters from that show — and we answered all of them, I might add," Rapp tells me. "Not a week goes by that I don't see a patient who saw that show and came here because of it."

Among those patients are Colin Sheehan and his brother, Gregory, from Queens, New York, across the East River from Manhattan. "I happened to be watching television, and I saw Dr. Rapp on *Donahue*," recalls their mother, Charlotte. "I said, 'My God, this is my kid!' I couldn't believe it. She described him to a T, complete to the red earlobes that I had to pack in ice because they would pain him so much. I contacted Dr. Rapp, and in 1989, when Colin was in third grade, we came here."

The years up to third grade were enough to make any young mother think twice about the joy of having kids. "When Colin was born he had severe colic," Charlotte recalls. "He would pull his knees to his chest and cry all the time. He was in agony. Then he didn't have a bowel movement for two days. So I called the doctor. He said, 'Don't worry. Everything's fine. When it's been four days, then worry.'

"I thought, 'Your child, you worry at four days. My child, I worry at two days.' Everything I learned in nursing school said newborns shouldn't be acting like this."

Thus began a harrowing journey for Charlotte, a part-time nurse, her husband, Joe, an anesthetist, and their two kids. "I didn't accept this," Charlotte says. "I kept going from doctor to doctor. I finally settled on one who put Colin on soy formula.

Up until this point they had only prescribed phenobarbital. Primarily for me." She laughs. "I was obviously a nervous mother."

As we talk in Rapp's waiting room, all around us kids are squawking, mothers fidgeting, nurses escorting anxious families into the office. Suddenly Colin appears at his mother's side. He's thirteen now, a dark-haired, pug-nosed, round-faced, slim and smallish junior high schooler.

"We have a problem," he says. "I'm starving!"

"Colin," Charlotte says. "Outta the bag take some fruit, get some grapes. Yeah, you need the sugar . . ."

Colin saunters back to the far end of the waiting room, reaches into the bag of food, starts munching on a handful of grapes, returns to his comic book. Next to him, Gregory, his ten-year-old brother, a Colin carbon copy except for his flaming red hair, does the same thing.

Charlotte laughs. "Yeah, yeah," she says to me. "They don't get brains until they're about twenty-one."

But back when Colin was born, it seemed unlikely that he would make it to thirteen, much less twenty-one. Even on the soy formula, Colin continued to suffer, spitting up like crazy. "We fed him every four hours, *not* on demand," says Charlotte. "If we fed him on demand, he had more colic. I didn't sleep at night until he was fifteen months of age. He was up all the time."

All this was only the beginning. By the time he was a toddler, Colin presented his family with a bundle of new problems. "He had constant sore throats," recalls Charlotte. "And whenever the grass was cut, he would become very irritable. Then, when he got older, about two, he would break out in temper tantrums like you wouldn't believe. Everybody would tell me that I wasn't disciplining him enough, but I knew something was wrong. But the pediatrician didn't agree with me."

Then came the headaches and strange infections — swollen glands, aching knees and legs — and endless rounds of antibiotics. Nothing helped. Colin went through a year and a half of allergy shots, for dust and mites. They didn't help. He saw a chiropractor. That didn't help. Then bad went to worse.

"By the third grade he started having multiple tics. Face, neck, arms, legs," remembers Charlotte. "It got so bad he couldn't walk. When he tried, he looked like Michael Jackson moon-walking. We went to pulmonologists, cardiologists, the whole gamut. And didn't get any answers. He wasn't growing that much, wasn't gaining weight. He was sick all the time. The temper tantrums were getting out of control."

So the Sheehans came all the way from Queens to see Doris Rapp. However, Rapp's treatment was at first only a modest success. "When she started testing Colin, we found out that he was a very difficult tester," says Charlotte. "There were so many symptoms, and his system had been so taxed for so long, that it was hard to find out what was wrong with him. Dr. Rapp had a hard time finding neutralizing doses. At the end of three days of testing she was extremely upset, because we went home with only five. But I was grateful, because that was five more than we had before."

One of those neutralizing doses was for beef. Another was for dairy products, another for potatoes, another for chlorine. And the last was a neutralizing dose for histamine itself. "It's a nonspecific way to treat an allergic reaction, just as aspirin is a nonspecific way to treat a headache," Rapp explains. "Regardless of the cause of a headache, aspirin often helps. Treatment with the correct neutralization dilution of histamine often relieves the allergic symptoms regardless of whether the cause is egg, grass pollen, or some other substance."

"So now he can eat his beef, and he can eat his potatoes," says Charlotte. And today the Sheehans are in Buffalo to retest the boys' reactions to foods. "We come up three, four times a year," Charlotte says. "Dr. Rapp retests their foods to make sure everything is okay."

A nurse carrying a clipboard and an oven timer escorts

Colin from the waiting room into the testing room. There a crowd of kids and parents surrounds a nurse stationed at a table covered by a mountain of vials of clear liquid. These are the provocation and neutralizing doses. All day long the testing goes on. Kids fearfully, tearfully, sometimes stoically bare their arms. Nurses wearily inject dose after dose after dose, wind their oven timers to seven minutes, and watch to see what happens. Now Colin takes his place at the table. What I've just seen on videotape prepares me for the worst. As it turns out, needlessly.

"Colin's not one of these kids who gets violent and runs around," says Charlotte. "That's why he can be hard to test — he doesn't draw your attention."

First Colin receives a provocation dose of chlorine. Soon his tics begin. And his eyes roll. But not too badly. Colin has come a long, long way. "There's no comparison with before," says Rapp. "Colin couldn't walk down the street, couldn't feed himself, he was twitching so badly when he first came in. Now he comes in, and many times I don't even see a tic."

After P/N doses of beef, rice, potato, and molds, Colin rests in the waiting room. Rapp appears for one of her periodic tours of the outer sanctum. "Look at those ears," she says, cheerfully. "Some nice red ears there."

And so it goes, for three days. During that time Colin receives close to twenty doses, and takes back with him to Queens a handful of new extracts for immunotherapy. "He got an overhaul," laughs Charlotte. "He got regreased and reoiled."

Rick Kiessig came away from his skin testing with *one hundred* extracts to take back to California. In fact, in the two weeks he was in Dallas he did little else but skin testing. "I'd get there at nine in the morning and leave at six-thirty at night," he says. "It was a lot of pokes in the arm." He laughs. "I figured I had come all the way to Dallas. Might as well take advantage of it."

Although he never carried on quite as dramatically as some of the kids in Rapp's videos, from time to time Kiessig found himself surprised by the intensity of his reactions — especially to his particular bugaboo, molds.

"My reactions were mostly wheals," he says. "But maybe ten out of the hundred times, I had bad symptoms. They found specific molds that made me so completely out of it I couldn't even talk. My brain just turned off. Then the neutralization doses brought me right back. I found out that molds are terrible for me."

Besides that, the skin tests showed Kiessig which foods caused him problems: milk, nuts, soy, pork, chicken, various fish and vegetables. And the center's nutritionist suggested a method of avoiding those foods. "They wait until you've completed the skin testing on the first round of basic foods," says Kiessig. "Then you have an appointment with the nutritionist. She gives you a book — makes you pay for it, actually — that breaks down the food by families and describes how to alternate those food families in a four-day rotation diet."

In his eyes, then, Rick's visit to Dallas was a success. "It had such a dramatic effect on my life," he says. "I learned how to turn off almost all my reactions with the extracts. I learned which things I could be near and which I should avoid. I've tried to adjust my environment to reflect those sensitivities to the extent I could. But I haven't yet been able to implement a rotation diet."

The rotation diet is another legacy from Theron Randolph, who himself borrowed it from others. Doris Rapp, too, employs the rotation diet as a way of testing the impact of various foods while simultaneously alleviating or even preventing reactions to them. The crux is alternating food groups every four days.

"It's very easy to follow," says Rapp. "You just pick a food family and eat it each day. For example, beef and milk go together. But you wouldn't have beef the next day. Maybe you'd have ham or pork. After that you could have turkey. Then after that you could have chicken, because even though they're both poultry, turkey and chicken are in different families. You could also add in tuna or different kinds of fish, because they're a different family." And fruits, vegetables, grains, and other foods line up in kind. The categories aren't always obvious or intuitive — the separation of chicken and turkey into different families is a prime example. Like Rea, Rapp provides her patients with a detailed chart of which foods go with which.

The idea is that once on the rotation diet, if your, or your child's, health or behavior deteriorates every fourth day, the odds are pretty good that a particular food is at fault. The diet is therefore a solid diagnostic tool. At the same time, the rotation is a modified version of avoidance, allowing the body to rid itself of problem foods. "We know that it takes four days for the food you eat to leave your body," says Rapp. "In that way, you don't overload your system. What's happening with a lot of people who have unrecognized sensitivities to food is that they might eat a food without realizing it. For example, corn is found in a tremendous number of products — soda, cereals, anything that's sweet-tasting has corn syrup. So if you have sensitivity to corn, you may be overloading your body with it. Whereas if you have corn only every four days, your body might start to control it without any kind of medical treatment. A lot of parents will put their child on a rotation diet, and pretty soon they'll see a child who is without learning problems or severe, violent reactions, the child they knew was inside there all the time."

But it can be tough for patients to incorporate the diet into their lives. If it's a chicken, rice, peas, cranberry sauce day, for example, it's chicken, rice, peas, and cranberry sauce *every meal* during the day. And the food is not your run-of-the-mill supermarket fare. Many MCS sufferers do best on high-quality foods, foods without hormones, antibiotics, preservatives. And meanwhile, patients complement the diet with regular injections of neutralizing extracts gleaned from the provocation-neutralization skin tests. Treatment for MCS can sometimes seem as exhausting as the malady itself.

For Colin, the diet and injections serve primarily to maintain the tolerance it has taken him so long to build up. "He's eating well," Charlotte says. "He's taking advanced science and math courses. He's turning out to be a very good student. He's really doing wonderfully."

Nevertheless, Charlotte is realistic. Colin *is* doing wonderfully, but his life may never approach what anyone would consider normal. "Between you and me," she tells me, "I'm really concerned. What about when he starts dating? He's going to run into all sorts of problems. That's when his heart is going to be broken."

"It's like walking on eggshells," Rapp says. "He has to be *very* careful. And he's reached an age where he's getting concerned about his future. His parents have a good house, and they stick to the diet, and his mom does all the cooking from scratch, and their whole life revolves around these two kids. But it's not easy."

But don't tell that to Colin. "My friends used to always try not to eat things I can't have in front of me. Now I can have half the things they have," he says. "And my new friends don't even know I have allergies. I can do sports, but I have to have a shot sometimes 'cause of the grass. My life used to be really far off, but now it's getting closer to everybody else's."

In June of 1994, five months after his first visit, Rick Kiessig returned to Dallas to sample another of Bill Rea's wares: heat therapy. As might be expected, it, too, is controversial.

"Heat therapy!" snorts Rea, as though it's the most common thing in the world. "I didn't come up with that. American Indians and Romans came up with it. Swedes and Finns and all those guys came up with it, okay? Randolph came up with it. But we adapted it. When I heard about it, I said, 'This makes sense, we've got to do it.'"

L. Ron Hubbard came up with it too. A science fiction writer and founder of the religious movement (some would say cult) scientology, Hubbard also was known for his work in drug rehabilitation. Rea's version of Hubbard's process is based on the premise that toxins accumulate in the body — specifically in the body's fat. If it were possible to reduce that accumulation, the result would be better health. The idea of heat therapy, then, is to get rid of toxins by literally sweating them out of you.

EHC-Dallas has two saunas, each maintained at 150°. In contrast to the wooden saunas most of us are familiar with, these saunas are made completely of ceramic tile — floor, ceiling, walls. The only wood — the benches — is untreated poplar, as the hardwood contains relatively little resin, which is a problem for some sensitive people. "We maintain a controlled environment," says Rea. "Think of some of the saunas you've been to. Some have cedar wood, with all its terpenes. Sweat from one person drips onto the benches, soaks in, then the next guy gets up there. Some saunas have carpeting. You call that bizarre? What happens when that carpet and all its chemicals heat up?

"We're very meticulous. We make people sit on towels, so they can take 'em out with 'em. That's because sometimes our patients are so sensitive they react to each other. Everything we've done is to try and cut down on pollution."

The regimen starts with exercise, then sauna, then massage, all of which is preceded by patients being given vitamin C, amino acids, and other supplements, including niacin, which dilates their blood vessels. Then it's onto the treadmills, ideally for twenty to thirty minutes, then, once they've started to work up a good sweat, into the saunas to finish the job. After that, a shower and a massage. The massage is supposed to further work out toxins from fatty tissues and into the bloodstream and gut, where they can be expelled. And then to the next go round, and the next. Ideally, patients do three saunas a day.

Some people I met in Dallas swear by the saunas. Others can hardly tolerate them, claiming that toxins pour out so fast that they get excruciating headaches or asthma attacks. For Kiessig, the effect was less pronounced, but enjoyable. "I really liked it," he says. "I worked my way up to forty-five minutes in there. Before you go in, your skin gets very itchy and hot, but inside, that largely goes away after five, ten minutes. You're supposed to drink water. There's a guy outside the sauna who will refill your glass. In forty-five minutes I could drink liters of water.

"By the end of my stay I could do two a day. They tend to wipe you out, but they feel wonderful. When I came home I went out and bought a commercial low-toxic sauna that we installed in the house. My wife gets a much bigger spike from it than I do. For her it's energizing. For me it's restful and relaxing. It's not a miracle cure, but I feel that long term it's going to be an important way for me to get toxics out of my system."

Kiessig did not experience the most ambitious — and to outsiders, perhaps most outlandish — of the center's testing and treatment facilities: the Environmental Control Unit, or ECU.

The idea of an ECU was Theron Randolph's. If exposure to foods and chemicals causes problems, why not eliminate that exposure and see what happens? In the early 1950s Randolph began testing the notion by appropriating a few hospital rooms, depositing his patients inside, and subjecting them to a four-day water fast in order to purge their systems of any possible contaminants. Then he tested them for allergies. "The experiment was a success," he wrote, "and certain foods and chemical allergies were diagnosed that simply could not have been found through any of the office procedures used at that time."

But Randolph began to realize that it wouldn't do simply to use any old hospital room. A much more controlled setting was necessary. In 1975, he took the final step, opening what he called an Ecology Unit in a separate section of a hospital in a Chicago suburb. Although he later moved the unit, he continued to operate it until 1986, when, to his everlasting consternation, faced with declining coverage by patients' insurance, he was forced to shut it down. "One by one, Medicare, governmental health insurance programs based on Medicare policies, and private insurance carriers followed suit and refused to reimburse patients for such stays. Few patients, of course, could afford the expense of an extended hospital stay on their own. By early 1986, there were simply not enough insured patients to make the unit viable. To my great distress, it was necessary to close."

Today Bill Rea's ECU is the only remaining facility of its kind in the country. It's a last resort. For the most part, only the very sickest people, people for whom other measures simply haven't worked, end up there. Located in a secluded wing on the top floor of Dallas's Tri+City Hospital, the unit consists of six rooms of two beds each. Its entrance is insulated from the rest of the hospital by a dead-air space sandwiched between two heavy glass doors. Pass through this airlock and you're in a clean, controlled world. Nothing from the main hospital — no odors, no toxins, no contaminated air — can cross this barrier. Nothing, that is, except what people bring in. So visitors are cautioned not to wear perfumes, synthetic clothing, or any other possible irritants, and to don hospital gowns before visiting patients inside.

The unit doesn't look like much, however. It was converted from an oldish, drab, gray hospital wing, and it still looks like an oldish, drab, gray hospital wing. "It's very simple, very plain," Rea says. "But I tell you, it works!"

The floor is tile, the walls tile and porcelain. No potentially irritating wood, fabrics, plastic, or rubber here, no fluorescent lights with their flicker and strong electromagnetic fields — the lighting in the rooms is from incandescent bulbs. The unit receives its own filtered water and filtered air. As in the center, each room's TV set is encased in a glass-front cabinet that blocks electromagnetic and vapor emissions. All clothing, bedding, and towels are made of cotton, silk, or linen. Meals are prepared in stainless steel or glass cookware and served in stainless steel or glass containers with stainless steel utensils. Food is organic, water comes from springs and is bottled in glass. It's about as pristine an environment as you can get.

"People say, 'Don't put me back on the other side,'" says Rea, laughing.

They may not feel that way early on, however. The first thing the ECU staff has to do is wean people from the contaminated life they've been living. These people have become accustomed to their environment; this so-called adaptation, or masking, is a crucial concept in environmental medicine. Rea defines it this way: "Adaptation is an acute survival mechanism in which the individual gets used to a constant toxic exposure in order to survive, at the same time suffering a long-term decrease in efficient functioning and perhaps longevity." In other words, when you're constantly exposed to an irritant — auto exhaust, for example, or coffee — after an initially strong reaction, you simply become used to it. Your body adapts to the constant assault. You become masked. After a while you can't even tell that anything bothers you. It's just that now you function a little less efficiently. You may suffer a nagging headache for no apparent reason, or a cold that just won't go away, or an unrelenting battle with fatigue or fuzziness. Those are the signs of your body's attempt to deal with the contamination, the trade-off it makes to survive. Better a low-grade malaise that lets you function than an acute reaction that knocks you for a loop. That's adaptation, or masking.

What Rea tries to do in the ECU is get rid of that veneer of tolerance. That way he can obtain an accurate picture of what's going on, rather than being fooled by the body's survival subterfuge. So the first thing patients are asked to do when entering the ECU is fast — three to four days of a water fast to clear their system. That, in combination with living in a clean, controlled environment, should be enough to remove the body's blinders — to de-mask, de-adapt. Here Jerry Ross's comments are particularly pertinent, because he's intimately familiar with the ECU from both sides. His entrée to environmental medicine was as a patient.

"Three or four days is not as long as Randolph recommended, but it's the best we can do," Ross says. "Because, candidly, insurance companies don't like paying for people sitting around in the hospital not doing anything. You're treating them, you truly are, but the insurance companies don't recognize that. You have to be doing something *to* patients — giving them an IV, for example. Then insurance companies will say, 'Well, sure, they have to be in the hospital to get an IV, that's fair.' But an IV may not be the best thing for them at all. It's quite ridiculous."

During the fasting–de-masking period, as the body clears itself, patients may literally go through withdrawal. Chronic headaches may grow unbearable. Joint pains can become excruciating. Melancholy may descend into depression. But all that is nothing compared to what Ross himself went through in 1986, when, reeling from chest and joint pains, with muscles burning from a reaction to what he later learned was dry-cleaning fluid that had contaminated the water supply of his hometown in Nova Scotia, he entered the ECU.

"I had been on an anticonvulsant medication from a neurologist in an effort to help control the neurological pain and all the burning," he recalls. "The medication did help, but when I went into the ECU I stopped taking it. And promptly had a grand mal seizure.

"It's called a rebound phenomenon. If you stop an anticonvulsant, and if you're unlucky, you'll have an electrical excitation as a rebound. That's what happened to me. During the seizure I broke a bone in my back. It was like going from the frying pan into the fire."

At the end of the de-masking withdrawal period, patients usually feel better — Ross did. In fact, they may feel much better, better than they have in months or years. Simply being free of what ails them can make a huge difference. The next step is to test their sensitivities. First, because some 90 percent of chemically sensitive people react to contaminants in water, the staff gives patients various kinds of bottled spring water.

"We give them different kinds to see which they can tolerate," Ross says. "Most people will tolerate a high-quality, glass-bottled, filtered water." That particular water is their baseline fluid for the balance of their stay in the ECU and thereafter.

Then it's on to foods. The staff presents new foods, one per meal, and observes the patients' reactions. If their symptoms return, that food is scratched from the list. And patients themselves become an integral part of the testing process, keeping a detailed log of their reactions.

Finally, patients are challenged with chemicals. Here's where things become especially interesting. These tests take place in small, phone booth–sized chambers made of glass and steel. While this "booth testing" is a staple in the ECU, it also takes place in the clinic itself, to supplement or reinforce results gleaned through skin testing. "It's not routine," Ross says. "In the clinic it's usually reserved for certain circumstances that require more rigorous proof than skin testing provides. If lawsuits are involved, for example. Less than five percent of our patients do booth testing. It's too time-consuming and expensive." Nevertheless, EHC-Dallas has done more than fifteen thousand of these challenges.

First the staff measures patients' vital signs and administers various mental-function tests. Then the patients climb into the booths, and there they stay for the next few hours while low doses of vaporized chemicals are piped in. "Each challenge lasts for fifteen minutes if the patient can tolerate that much exposure," explains Ross. "They can abort any time they wish."

Patients don't know in advance which chemical is coming — it's a single-blinded test. Occasionally no chemical is presented at all — the only thing piped into the booth is a placebo of vaporized water or saline solution. Sometimes neither the patient nor the person giving the test knows what's coming. That's a double-blinded test, the most objective procedure possible. To discover what's what, a code must be broken afterward. If patients experience a reaction, or if a repeat of the vital signs and mental tests now reveal significant fluctuations, odds are that that particular chemical is something to be avoided.

"I learned a great deal from booth testing," says Ross. "I learned I was sensitive to formaldehyde, phenol, and a few other chemicals. Then I was exposed to the dry-cleaning fluid. I was convinced that it was a placebo, because I couldn't smell anything. But within about an hour I couldn't think. I couldn't even reproduce little diagrams. I broke out in a rash. My blood pressure went down. I went all sweaty. My joint pains came back. I got my brain fog. I really felt like an idiot. When we broke the code, lo and behold, it was the dry-cleaning fluid.

"I went home with knowledge — knowledge about what I was sensitive to, knowledge of how to make changes. I went home with shots that helped to make me less sensitive. I went home on a rotation diet. And I realized that with what I had learned I was not going to be content going back to the same kind of medicine — seeing a lot of runny noses and such, just sort of pushing medication. I wanted to try to help some of the people like me who were being missed in the regular medical community. So I went into environmental medicine."

Avoidance, nutritional therapy, immunotherapy, heat therapy — these are the heart of the EHC-Dallas approach to multiple chemical sensitivity. But there's more, both on the diagnostic and treatment side. For example, Rea and his colleagues use a variety of high-tech tests to identify and confirm the presence of chemical sensitivity. One is called pupilography. By measuring the response of the eye's pupils to a flash of light, they claim it's possible to detect the kind of damage to the autonomic nervous system frequently found in MCS patients. The change in the pupil's size, the speed of contraction and dilation, and the time the pupil takes to recover to normal are usually consistent in any individual. The pupils of people with MCS, on the other hand, tend to react erratically. The machine used to take these measurements is called a binocular iriscorder and was developed by Japanese research colleagues of Rea's, one of whom busily experiments with his device in an office at the center.

Another test involves single photon emission tomography, or SPECT. A new brain-imaging technique much like CAT and PET scans, SPECT tracks the flow of blood into the brain and the brain's ability to utilize that blood. "You can actually differentiate patterns of neurotoxicity," says Rea. "You take a scan of a patient who has a neurotoxic pattern of the brain, then you get him better, then you give him of whiff or two of the chemical that you know he's sensitive to, okay? Then you go ahead and do another scan on him — he'll show the toxic pattern again."

The image derived from a SPECT scan resembles a multicolored jewel, with its computer-generated hues conveying information about the brain it pictures. In the case of normal uptake of blood, red and white predominate. Abnormal perfusion is denoted by yellow, green, and blue. Rea's patients often display a salt-and-pepper pattern that he's come to recognize as a tip-off for neurological damage.

"With most of the patients we do a scan as confirmation," he says. "We've got it down to where we can diagnose things in the clinic pretty good. We can tell the ones that are going to have a positive SPECT scan. So we just use it as backup. For legal cases, anybody who's in doubt." Of the patients Rea has scanned, 90 percent show neurological damage.

Other treatments at the center include various methods of boosting the immune system. "I like to call 'em tolerance modulators," says Rea. One of those requires injecting into patients an extract of healthy white blood cells gleaned from the patients themselves. "You can take white cells from patients, grow them in tissue culture, get 'em robust, and inject them back. It boosts the immune system, stops infection, boosts energy, and helps keep away immune depression. We call it an autogenous vaccine."

So far Rick Kiessig likes the results of the immune-system booster. "It has a very slow and subtle effect, but what I and others have noticed is that if we get off it, a month to six weeks later we feel absolutely awful. I've been on it since July of 'ninety-five. My wife started in January."

Rea, too, has sampled the technique. In fact, in an attempt to deal with his own sensitivities, he's tried just about everything the clinic has to offer. "I take food shots for corn, beef, sugar, pork, and wheat. Wheat and corn bother me the most. I try to eat organic food all the time. I don't drink or smoke. Don't do drugs. Supplements? Sure, you bet. I do sauna sometimes. I've done the autogenous stuff." He laughs. "I'm the guinea pig in this clinic."

Finally — and this approach stems from the experiences that prompted Rea to tackle the problem of MCS in the first place — the center sometimes recommends surgery. Not to remove body parts, but rather to rid the body of internal sources of contamination: prostheses, synthetic mesh used to reinforce incisions, even silver/mercury tooth fillings. The reasoning here is that if petroleum-derived products like plastic, and metals like mercury can irritate on the outside, imagine what they might be doing to you internally.

"If prosthetic devices can be taken out, we take 'em out," Rea says. "We change heart valves for people. We've been taking out a lot of hernia mesh. It's a synthetic. We do quite a lot of surgery like that, because it really does help people."

If people can afford such treatments. Treatment for MCS is not cheap, and insurance coverage is at best problematic — and not only for stays in the environmental control unit. "You can't expect insurance companies to pay for unproven treatment," says a physician who treats MCS patients. And often they don't.

The Kiessig family can't count on insurance. "These people are expensive, and insurance doesn't pay for everything," says Lynne Kiessig. For example, Rick's initial two-week stay at EHC-Dallas came to some $5,500 — $3,000 for lab work and $2,500 for office visits and skin testing. And that doesn't cover lodging, food, or transportation from California to Texas. "My husband's disability insurance should have paid a fair amount of money — they never came through," Lynne says. "But we did get some from our comprehensive health policy."

The family's policy promises to pay 80 percent of legitimate health expenses — for Rick's treatments, however, it paid about 40 percent. (The center offers a special rate for those relying on Medicare, which, in many patients' experience, has been more willing to cover costs than private insurance carriers have.)

The Sheehan family also has felt the brunt. Colin's and Gregory's three days of testing with Doris Rapp costs about $1,200 — for each child. "That's not counting airfare or staying at a Residence Inn," says Charlotte Sheehan. "And she's not expensive compared to others." These days the Sheehans' Blue Cross–Blue Shield pays for 80 percent of the cost of their periodic visits, and perhaps a third of the cost of extracts, which can run in the neighborhood of $400 per session. But it wasn't always like this.

"For a while, they wouldn't pay at all," Charlotte says. "My husband was called up during the Gulf War, and I had to go back to work. Blue Cross held up payments for about a year until I threatened legal action. Subsequently they paid."

But they don't pay for the Sheehans' Manhattan environmental doc. "Sometimes Colin is so up and down that we can't afford to keep going back to Buffalo. Besides, we need somebody for extract supplements. But they won't pay." Charlotte laughs — the weary laugh of someone who has become resigned to her fate. "These boys are the summer house we were going to buy in North Carolina, our new cars, our summer vacations. Our accountant looks at our bills and gets hysterical laughing."

All of it — the surgery, the immune boosters, the rotation diets, the vitamin and mineral supplementation, the immunotherapy shots, the avoidance — all of it is aimed at one overriding goal: to help patients better handle the stress visited upon them by the environment.

"Think of a patient as a rain barrel," says Ross. "The water in the barrel is the total load of environmental pollutants that the body must cope with. Then along comes some other source of stress. But the barrel can't hold it, and it pours out. The overflow represents a health problem. The load goes too high, something has to give, and you get sick."

This concept of "total load" is central to environmental docs' attempts to come to grips with MCS. And with a disease that so far has defied definitive explanation, this concept may be as good as any.

"Total load is the sum total of all the various kinds of stressors that our bodies have to contend with," says Ross. "One component is the accumulation of toxic chemicals in the body, but it's only one. Foods are another. In fact, of all the materials that we receive from outside that our bodies have to deal with, foods are by far the most important. Other things include microbes — they're part of the total load. Our electromagnetic milieu is part of the total load. Stress — psychosocial forces are part of the total load. And a very important part of the total load is your genetic endowment — you're stuck with that. Total load is the sum total of all the stuff you have to digest, cough or sneeze out, metabolize in some way, detoxify, deal with."

In other words, the water in the barrel represents the impact of the entire environment: physical, psychological, emotional. We are an integrated organism, Ross is saying. Any one stressor, any one incitant, affects the whole. That is total load. Given that concept, then, the task is to define its particulars and figure out how to manage them.

"You have to ask yourself this vital question: 'What caused the overflow?'" Ross says. "Modern medicine says, 'Well, some stuff just poured into the barrel and that caused the overflow.' But that doesn't help at all. Just slapping a Band-Aid on the immediate problem does no good. The answer is, 'All the other stuff *already in the barrel* contributed to the overflow as well.'

"For example, if you have a certain amount of ongoing chemical exposure, you may be able to adapt to that. But have a few other things happen — like a big argument with your boss, or infection with a virus, or staying up too late and not getting enough sleep — then the barrel can overflow."

"Supposing, then, by various means — dietary avoidance, environmental cleanup with air filters, better nutrition, psychological support, whatever — you get the level of the water down to halfway in the barrel. Then along comes some other stressor, and it doesn't overload you. It doesn't make you sick.

"So all the stuff we do in environmental medicine can be boiled down to four simple words: *lower the total load.*"

The concept seems simple enough, but the sheer variety of what's going on at EHC-Dallas can make your head spin. As I wander through the clinic talking to physicians, staff, and patients, I begin to get the idea that, emptying the barrel notwithstanding, when it comes to MCS, anything goes. Got a bright idea? Give it a shot. What has anyone got to lose?

"Sounds like what you're doing here is flying by the seat of your pants," I remark to Rea, none too delicately.

He doesn't bat an eye. "What is science, anyhow? You have an idea, and you think the idea is going to work, and you try it and see if it works. Then you substantiate it. That's what we do. We've always published. We've always shown the data.

"Besides, all the stuff we've done is so sound medically. For God's sake, avoidance has been around for how long? We've been washing wounds for a hundred years — that's avoidance therapy, okay? Quarantines for TB — that's avoidance therapy. Nutritional therapy has been around forever.

"What we're doing is just common sense."

Chapter **4**

All in Their Heads

OH YEAH?

Most physicians would contend that all that talk, all those treatments, all that "reducing the total load" business — all that — is bunk. *Something* is happening to these people — *that* everyone acknowledges. It is disagreement over the roots of that something, the mechanisms driving it, and the methods of treating it that causes conflict. After all, one of the tenets of orthodox medical training is that the more symptoms, the less likely a patient has a bona fide disease. Thus the official position taken by the American Medical Association: "Based on a lack of solid scientific data, the Council on Scientific Affairs of the American Medical Association cannot affirm that multiple chemical sensitivity syndrome (MCSS) exists as a recognized clinical entity."

Moreover, many of the symptoms these people display — brain fog, confusion, disorientation — are psychological in nature. Maybe MCS is a psychogenic problem. Maybe it's all in their heads.

* * *

A number of mainstream physicians share this opinion. Typical are the sentiments of University of Iowa College of Medicine psychiatrist Donald Black. "It's my belief that people diagnosed as having environmental illness in most cases do have something wrong: a garden variety emotional disorder."

Black's conclusion is the aftermath of an unforeseen encounter with a patient diagnosed as suffering from hypersensitivity to a common irritant. While screening prospective volunteers for a study of obsessive-compulsive disorder, he happened to interview a thirty-five-year-old woman who told him that her doctor attributed her compulsion to constantly wash her hands to an overgrowth in her body of candida yeast. In other words, her bizarre behavior was the result of an allergic reaction to a yeast infection. That struck Black as dubious. "There aren't many patients who tell me that a previous doctor has explained their obsessive-compulsive disorder in terms of chronic yeast disease. The story sounded so bizarre that I thought I'd research it further."

He and his colleagues recruited twenty-six people who had been diagnosed with MCS, psychologically evaluated them, and compared their personality profiles with those of controls, forty-six "normal" people. The result was that a whopping 65 percent of the MCS patients, as compared to only 28 percent of the controls, exhibited evidence of major mental disorders. "We conclude that patients receiving this diagnosis may have one or more commonly recognized psychiatric disorders that could explain some or all of their symptoms," the team wrote. In other words, MCS is a psychiatric disease. And so entrenched are their mental problems, Black doubts these people are even treatable. "It's virtually impossible to deprogram them. I wouldn't even attempt it."

John Selner does all the time. A Denver allergist and respiratory specialist, Selner, who works with psychologist Herman

Staudenmayer, claims that he can cure most of his patients by deprogramming them to eliminate their "false" beliefs. "We can help fifty to seventy-five percent of patients who are amenable to therapy," he says. "'Amenable' — that's the key. They have to accept where they are and try to change. You have to wean them away from an 'I can't handle anything' sort of attitude. But it takes time. I'm talking about long-term therapy. I don't mean a week either. Six months to a year in some people for them to really break through.

"Our treatment is traditional psychotherapy combined with other different kinds of approaches," he explains. "Traditional talk psychotherapy usually doesn't work with these people initially. So we do a lot of work with self-regulation, relaxation, biofeedback. Get these people's symptoms under control first, then we talk about what might have caused them. We're just taking what other schools of psychotherapy have shown to work and combining them in another way."

No one is more qualified than Selner to make such a statement. If Bill Rea is the most prominent environmental physician seeing MCS patients, Selner is the most prominent mainstream allergist. The first time he and I talked was after office hours, in a Mexican bar across the street from his Denver clinic. A self-assured sixty-one-year-old with short-cropped gray hair, a flattish, weathered face, and a soft-spoken, nasal delivery, Selner (who goes by "Jack") tends to describe his experiences in rambling monologues. "I was visiting at the University of Arizona in 1975," he tells me. "I was talking to the guy running the allergy department down there, and he said, 'Wonder if you'd like to go out to the desert with me? There's a woman who has some very peculiar symptoms. She can't come in to be examined, so I'm going out to see her. Do you want to come along?'"

Selner accompanied his friend. What he saw was a forty-five-year-old woman eking out a hermit's existence in a 7- by 12-foot trailer. The inside of the trailer was gloomy, almost impenetrable. She kept it darkened, she explained, because she couldn't stand the sun's ultraviolet rays. A Seeing Eye dog led her around. Her telephone was covered with aluminum foil so she didn't have to touch plastic. She complained of reactions to a variety of foods and chemicals and was not willing to travel into Tucson for medical tests because she'd have to pass beneath magnetic fields generated by power lines.

"I was fascinated by this lady," Selner says. "I saw things that didn't make a lot of sense. She had actually been licensed to have a dog for the blind help her make her way around the darkened trailer, but how the dog could see well enough to lead her was a mystery. And the thing that struck me was, she was highly tanned. If she had to stay inside most of the time because of ultraviolet rays, how did she get to be so tanned? It made no sense."

When Selner returned to town, he dug into the woman's case. He found that she had seen a number of doctors who had performed a number of examinations and lab tests and had found nothing wrong with her. She had undergone years of drug therapy and psychotherapy, also with no success. Finally, the woman had gone to a clinical ecologist, and finally she had received a diagnosis: "classical ecologic disease." Provocation-neutralization tests unearthed sensitivities to a variety of foods and chemicals. Blood tests showed abnormal levels of white blood cells, the prime disease fighters of the body's immune system. "The patient was declared allergic to the twentieth century," says Selner.

But when he went over the data, Selner could find no abnormal white blood cell counts. He was similarly unconvinced by the P/N conclusions. And he was astounded that the environmental doctor hadn't considered her psychiatric history a possible contributing factor in her illness. The man had simply declared her to be suffering from MCS. Selner felt that was a crime. "The conclusion of the clinical ecologist and accompanying recommendations seemed to represent a self-fulfilling prophecy, reinforcing her belief system, which protected her from facing the reality of psychiatric illness."

In Selner's opinion this woman didn't suffer environmental illness; rather, she was unstable, unreliable, badly in need of psychiatric help. "I saw a desperate human being," he says.

With that, he was hooked on the phenomenon of multiple chemical sensitivity. So hooked that in 1976 he paid a visit to the Environmental Health Center in Dallas. "I went down to take a look at Bill Rea's place," Selner says. "I saw somebody devoting himself to this problem. But there were a lot of contradictions. One was his lack of controls in his procedures. And I saw some people I thought were serious psychiatric cases. They should have been in a different setting. It was worrisome."

But one aspect of Rea's operation about which Selner had no reservations was his Environmental Control Unit. "I decided to try to duplicate their facility — even make it more strictly controlled — in Denver." In 1979, in collaboration with Theron Randolph's former trainee, environmental physician Kendall Gerdes, Selner opened his own ECU in Denver's large Presbyterian–St. Luke's Medical Center.

The project was ambitious but short-lived. It folded in 1984. The reasons why vary depending on who's doing the talking. First, there's Rea's version of the story. As might be expected in a head-to-head encounter of two strong personalities used to being in control, he and Selner do not get along. "I have no relationship with him," Selner says curtly. "We had a philosophical difference of opinion." "You'll get a lot of misinformation from Jack Selner," Rea told me in Dallas. "Jack came down and spent two and a half hours with me one Sunday afternoon. He became an instant expert on our ECU. But he couldn't make his unit run. He didn't understand it."

For his part, Selner blames the demise of his ECU on the economic realities of running a hospital. "The hospital people were looking for something better than a one-on-one operation." He shakes his head sadly. "If I had used my head back then, I would've gone to people who run universities and said, 'I want you to take over this facility. We'll run it — *you* get us the funds.' I think that would've worked.

"If we could have kept it alive, we could've been way ahead of answering these questions about MCS, and not be floating around with nobody coming up with anything satisfactory to anybody. It's an incredible shame what happened there.

"What we've done since is take everything we did in the ECU and put it on an outpatient basis and say, 'This may not be ideal by some people's vision of how things should be done, but it's the best we can do. We're gonna try to approach it from a different point of view.' And that's what we've been doing since."

A crucial part of Selner's "different" approach involves psychological therapy. That's where Herman Staudenmayer comes in. It's doubtful that there's a team anywhere like allergist Selner and psychologist Staudenmayer. Staudenmayer's office is in the basement of Selner's allergy complex. To the left a large leather couch, to the right Staudenmayer's desk. Diplomas and certificates adorn the wall. And there at the desk sits Staudenmayer. Fifty-one years old, suit and tie, bald head, thick glasses, mustache and goatee, a faint German accent — the psychologist of your dreams. MCS patients start upstairs with Selner for traditional allergy testing and other physiological examinations; often they find themselves finishing downstairs with Staudenmayer.

"There are several processes that are working here," he tells me. "The first one, the one I find most interesting, is the internal psychodynamics of the individual." Staudenmayer uses terms like "internal psychodynamics" and "iatrogenic," which means "induced by the physician." He's also fond of saying things like, "if you look at the history," and "in reviewing the literature . . ." They're an interesting duo, the rough-and-ready Selner, and Staudenmayer, the academic. In this case, the academic has had a strong influence on the clinician.

"The way I would characterize the situation is that there are many people who would like to project their misery onto something," Staudenmayer explains. "Through an appraisal process they identify an external, environmental issue. There's a long history of this. It could be environmental chemicals, it could be sugar, it could be candida . . . the list is endless. Those are the people who get attracted to MCS."

Indeed, there is a long history of vague, unsubstantiated illness marked by the very symptoms suffered by people with MCS. "There are several famous figures who had such illness," Staudenmayer says. "Florence Nightingale, the nurse, William James, the psychologist, Proust, the writer." The case of the turn-of-the-century French novelist Marcel Proust is particularly striking. He lived the last years of his life secluded in a cork-lined room so as to protect himself from dangers of the outside environment. His letters contain passages imploring visiting friends to refrain from wearing perfume or he'll never be able to see them again.

Not all historical manifestations of this illness focused on the environment, however. A case in point is the disease theory called autointoxication or self-poisoning. "It was a major mainstream medical proposition around the turn of the century — in fact, there were major operations done for it," says Ronald Gots, a physician-pharmacologist based outside Washington, D.C., who has written on the similarities between autointoxication and MCS.

The theory originated with a nineteenth-century French scientist named Frantz Glenard, who in 1886 wrote about a condition known as neuroesthenia, which was marked by fatigue, headaches, stomach pain, decreased appetite, a feeling of fogginess — exactly the same symptoms as MCS — and which was thought to be caused by the collapse of the digestive organs. By the turn of the century, numerous books and nearly a thousand articles had been written about the problem, with another thousand to come in the next decade. By this time, however, the cause of the malady had been broadened to emphasize the involvement of intestinal toxins, which supposedly were being produced at a rate exceeding the ability of the liver and kidneys to clear them.

What to do about the problem? "A London surgeon named Sir William Arbuthnot Lane taught people to perform all sorts of major operations," says Gots. This approach was justified by the recently invented X-ray machine, which revealed all sorts of misplaced, missized, and misshaped stomachs, intestines, and colons — all perfectly normal but thought to be evidence of autointoxication and the collapse of organs. So entire colons were removed, stomachs were taken away, "intestinal kinks" were unkinked, organs were stitched to the abdominal wall, adhesions were cut loose. And less catastrophic measures such as laxatives, purgatives, and enemas to remove toxins were also employed.

For Gots, MCS is this era's incarnation of autointoxication. The symptoms of both "diseases" are similar ("assigned diagnostic names and used repeatedly over the years to round out syndromes born of ignorance and doomed to oblivion," he writes), and both reflect, as in a distorted, funhouse mirror, the emerging knowledge of the times. At the turn of the century details about the workings of the digestive system were just coming to light; that information, and misinformation, was applied to explain autointoxication. Today we are discovering the vast influence of the environment in our lives, and so, based on our incomplete understanding, we blame the world around us for our problems. Autointoxication and MCS are born of similar misguided rationalization.

"It's a phenomenon that has been around for quite a while in various guises — no question about it," Gots exclaims. "These are people who, for a variety of reasons, don't function well and, usually at a subconscious level, are looking for some explanation for their problems. And they find it. At the turn of the century it was in intestinal malfunction. Now it's in environmental chemicals." Historically, these "diseases" have flourished until medical science develops to the point that it can disprove them. A similar fate, Gots feels, awaits MCS.

Herman Staudenmayer also sees the need to project problems onto something else as the first step in the onset of MCS. "Then there is, on the other end, the iatrogenic influence, which preys upon that vulnerability," he says. "These are the clinical ecology quack types, who are taking advantage of the situation. It is the induction of a false belief, for a variety of motives." In other words, the unfortunate influence of doctors who convince patients that the cause of their problems is the environment is the second step in Staudenmayer's explanation for the onset of MCS.

"The third factor is more of what typically happens in mass psychogenic illness — mutual reinforcement, through principles of contagion and spreading," Staudenmayer explains. "People talk to one another, commiserate with one another, and the disease spreads. When you review the literature concerning psychogenic illness you see that the time course doesn't quite fit what we call MCS. Spreading typically goes on in industrial sites, factories usually, where it happens in a matter of hours or days. There's a culmination and a quick resolution. It's all in the same environment. That's typically the example in the literature, but it doesn't mean it's limited to that.

"The most fascinating study I've ever seen concerns a town on the east coast. One day a guy went into the hall of records: 'My God, they've built this town on a toxic dump site.' All of a sudden everybody in town was getting sick. Doctors reported it to the Centers for Disease Control. They thought they had an epidemic. Until somebody looked at the records again and said, 'What is this nonsense?' The name of the town was the same as another town in another state where there actually was a toxic dump site. There was no toxic dump site here. The guy had gotten the wrong town. Suddenly everybody got well."

People who project their miseries onto the environment, physicians who reinforce the connection, and the power of mass psychogenic suggestion, the "misery loves company" phenomenon — for Staudenmayer and Selner, these are the steps leading to MCS.

But there's more to it than that. Why are people so miserable that they must attribute their problems to something other than themselves? Why are they so vulnerable to the influence of doctors and the power of suggestion? Those questions lead to the most startling facet of Staudenmayer and Selner's rationale concerning the origins of MCS. MCS, they contend, is the result of childhood abuse — in particular, sexual abuse.

Selner and Staudenmayer arrived at this disconcerting conclusion as a result of a study they conducted with sixty-three patients who professed to suffer from MCS. They subjected approximately half these patients to psychotherapy and found that compared to a control group with similar complaints but no suspicions of chemical exposure, the prevalence of physical and sexual childhood abuse was unusually high.

"It doesn't necessarily have to be sexual," says Staudenmayer. "There are other forms of conflicts and problems that are repressed. But sexual abuse was the most dramatic. It was in the fifty, sixty percent range. The reason that sexual abuse in childhood is so devastating is probably because of the horrifying psychological effects of terror. Being forced, being controlled. This gives a kind of abuse that is not one incident. This is chronic. And there's physical pain associated with it. There's threat. These people report unbelievable things."

As a case in point, the partners tell the story of one of their patients, a forty-five-year-old woman who worked in a newspaper office. Before coming to Selner and Staudenmayer she had been diagnosed as allergic to phenol, formaldehyde, glycerol, tricholoethane, chlorine, newsprint, and ethanol — with the result that her teeth chattered, she stammered when she spoke, and she suffered weakness, tremors on the right side of her body, sleep disorders, depression, cognitive problems. She was a mess.

As a prelude to testing the woman's sensitivity by exposing her to air containing formaldehyde and other chemicals, Selner and Staudenmayer placed her in an isolation chamber and pumped in clean air for half an hour. To their surprise, the woman responded as though she had been exposed to the chemicals. "This resulted in reproduction of her presenting symptoms, particularly tremor, weakness, and speech difficulties," they wrote in their report. They explained to her that sometimes patients react as she had simply because they anticipate how miserable they are going to feel and, sure enough, behave accordingly. Then the physicians gave the woman another dose of clean air. This time she developed none of the symptoms. But when they repeated the experiment one more time, again bathing her in clean air, she began trembling and stammering as before. It was clear that something was going on that had nothing to do with exposure to chemicals.

It took two subsequent years of psychotherapy to discover what that something was. The woman's father and older brother had abused her and other family members, both sexually and physically. For example, the woman's father once dipped an electric cord into a bathtub where she and her brother were bathing. The symptoms of electric shock that she experienced then — flushing, shaking, trembling — were similar to the so-called MCS symptoms that she developed much later. Another time her father forced her to swallow photo processing chemicals. Her nausea and vomiting then were much like her nausea and vomiting as an adult. "It appears that many, if not all, of the patient's symptoms were psychophysiologic reactions traceable to specific abuse scenarios, but projected onto the environment," the team wrote.

Slowly, through psychotherapy, the woman came to understand her feelings that "the world was not a safe place to live." And, claim Selner and Staudenmayer, she began to recognize that she had *learned* to suffer her myriad symptoms. The problem did not spring from the outside world — it came from within. One therapy session stands out. While remembering a traumatic incident, the woman began to tremble and hyperventilate. She blamed the Naugahyde of the couch she was sitting on. But the couch wasn't Naugahyde — it was leather. Rather than being assailed by the environment, she was suffering because of her memories. "Today she can sit on that couch and laugh about this episode," says Staudenmayer. And she's not the only one. Seventy-five percent of the patients in the study learned to handle their various symptoms through psychotherapy.

As I listen, I begin to wonder. Estimates suggest that the number of Americans claiming increased allergic sensitivity to chemicals is in the range of fiftieth percent of the population, at the least. That's a lot of people. "Is there enough childhood sexual abuse around to account for them all?" I ask.

Both Selner and Staudenmayer nod their heads vigorously. "It's a real difficult exercise in epidemiology," Staudenmayer says. "How do you define 'abuse'? How do you get people to tell the truth? Estimates of father-daughter incest range from eight percent to twenty-five percent. And that would be defined as penetration, only the severest form. Father-with-daughter abuse provides the best statistics available. But it doesn't have to be. Some of these instances are transgenerational. The numbers are higher than anything you'd ever want to imagine."

"Is it increasing?" I ask.

"Who knows?" Staudenmayer answers. "How do you make such an assessment? As recently as the late seventies the psychiatric community basically ignored the problem because the teachings of the psychodynamic tradition were that memories of sexual abuse was the fantasy of the child. But the paradigm shifted, starting in the late seventies. Today the psychoanalytic community has come out with some definitive papers acknowledging there was a mistake."

"These people are helpless, hopeless, with no place to go," says Selner. "They're screaming for some kind of assistance."

"And many, if you try to help them, they'll turn on you. They'll make *you* the victim of their madness," Staudenmayer says. "These are the ones about whom every textbook of psychiatry says, 'Be careful!' They're treatable but don't get near them — that's a catchword in the profession. Many of the MCS people are that type. We've treated at least a hundred of these very severe personality disorders, the potentially dangerous ones."

"Have any of these patients ever turned on you?" I ask.

"There was this one particular patient," Selner recalls. "The first time we saw her she was in the environmental unit. I was walking down the hall, and she was being combative with an orderly. I didn't know this person, never met her. I said something benign like, 'I'm sure it can't be that bad . . .' and *bang!* I got clobbered, and I went down! She floored me." He laughs and rubs his chin.

"After treatment she was eventually able to take a job with a chemistry laboratory — this was a chemically sensitive person! — and do a lot of very positive things. But I'm not about to say that one of these days she won't cold-cock somebody on the street who gets in her face."

"We're talking about people who were able to recognize that their beliefs were false beliefs and were able to move on to deal with the psychological issues," says Staudenmayer. "It does not mean that they were cured of their psychological problems. They addressed them and became functional, but I'm not so sure that anybody ever really recovers from that kind of history of trauma."

"How long before they're functional?" I ask.

"That's highly individual," Staudenmayer says. "Years sometimes."

"One last question," I say. "Up to eighty percent of people with MCS are women. Why?"

Staudenmayer answers. "I'm speculating — we're reduced to speculation at this point — that it's because of the much higher incidence of abuse among women than men. One of the confounding problems with abuse in men is that as adults they tend to act out violently and wind up in prison. And that's a black hole, because there's no information coming back in terms of their psychological status."

"I think it's tied up in hormonal influence," Selner says. "Think about the incredible effect that estrogen has in determining everything from the type of hair you have on your head to the texture of your skin, odors, the resiliency of various tissues, and on and on and on. Think about the changes in women associated with their periods — profound PMS, for example, which I don't think anybody argues isn't real. All that has to do with something peculiar to women. I've had young gals whose first significant asthma problem comes with menarche. They start having periods, and *wham!* — they start having asthma. You see women who have asthma become menopausal and stop having it. Women on birth control pills who are having trouble with asthma stop having it when they come off, or the opposite. Is this the kind of thing that results in what people call MCS? Who knows? It bothers the hell out of me. What do we know about estrogen, and progesterone, and the potential for their having a major influence on why women might be more susceptible to whatever this is?"

"There are many unknowns in MCS," says Staudenmayer. "Alluding to those unknowns as if you had an explanation is arrogance."

It's just such arrogance that mainstream physicians attribute to environmental docs' approach to the problem. Arrogance plus ineptness. For part and parcel of their conviction that MCS is a psychogenic problem is mainstream doctors' distrust of alternative theories to explain the disorder and alternative ways to treat it.

"The major techniques used by the clinical ecologists are controversial and unproven," states the American Academy of Allergy and Immunology. "There are no immunologic data to support the dogma of clinical ecologists. Clinical ecology . . . is an unproven and experimental methodology."

For example, what about total body load, the idea of the body's barrel filling with environmental incitants? "It makes no sense, none at all," declares Michael Straight, a former Centers for Disease Control toxicology and emergency medicine expert now practicing in Selner's clinic. "The body is a terrific eliminator of toxins. That's why you have a liver and kidneys. They work very well."

"It's testimony to the shortsightedness of individuals who really believe that your defense mechanisms have major limitations," adds Selner. "It just doesn't make sense that you conveniently have one more drop in the barrel, and all of a sudden you're sick."

"I'm pretty well convinced there are no true immune parameters that are affected by exposure to chemicals," says Straight. "I have looked for years hoping to find some and have not, outside of occupational high-level exposures. But for the average resident near a typical hazardous waste dump or Superfund site, or for the MCS population, I haven't seen any immune abnormalities that weren't a function of a lab report that is setting the test point for abnormalities so ridiculously low that the general population would flunk that test."

These mainstream docs are waiting to be shown. They're waiting for some kind of convincing evidence that illustrates the purported rise in contamination in the body. "I could see an instance where someone becomes very ill, or goes on a fast and loses a lot of weight, and pesticides stored in fat move into the bloodstream, raising pesticide levels in your blood," says Straight. "In that kind of situation you might argue that you can overwhelm the detoxification capacity of your body. However, there are a lot of problems with the blood tests these people use to see how well the immune apparatus is working. They're usually done by dubious labs with quality control that doesn't seem to exist. Until they're done in a reasonably controlled manner, among people with and without symptoms, so we get a database of normals to compare with, I don't know how to interpret those tests."

Another debatable tenet of environmental medicine is masking, or adaptation. "It's just an extension of a known phenomenon," Selner says. "Adaptation occurs when you walk into a room and smell an odor. The longer you're there, the harder it is to detect it. That's a natural kind of thing. But this elaborate scheme — I have trouble with that. It manages to explain *anything* you see. It's very convenient. Except there's no evidence that it's a model that can be demonstrated."

So little regard does Selner have for the concept, in his clinic's own chamber challenges, he and his colleagues don't even think of de-masking their patients. "We find that it really does not occur," says Straight. "People react right off the street."

Sick building syndrome is yet another suspect concept. Alan Hedge from the Department of Design and Environmental Analysis at Cornell has studied the phenomenon. He considers the most famous example, the EPA brouhaha, a "fiasco."

"All the analyses done on that building have failed to find that there was ever a significant risk to anybody," he says.

Michael Straight agrees. He thinks that Waterside Mall's ventilation system was almost certainly at fault, but that it's unlikely it caused any lasting problems. Something else was at work there.

"I've been in that building a lot," he says. "It's stuffy. I can imagine that having a week or two's worth of high-level exposure because the ventilation just couldn't get the air out of there probably did cause a lot of irritation. Plus it's a notoriously unpleasant place to be. It's in the middle of downtown D.C., with little block rooms, thousands of people swarming around there, overworked, underpaid. People are unhappy, under a lot of stress. I think what happened is that a response became triggered every time people smelled something in there."

What probably happened, then, is a dramatic instance of mass psychogenic hysteria. "One of the things about the design of many modern buildings is that the spaces have been built to facilitate communication," Hedge says. "What that means is that the social-political dynamic that causes the spread of complaints can be accelerated in many of these buildings."

As an example, Hedge tells the story of a building in Anchorage, Alaska, that eventually had to be evacuated. "It started with a problem of turf cutting outside the building. One employee reported odor problems and some difficulty in breathing. This employee was then moved out of her own office into another part of the building, into an office with two men and two women. Within two weeks two of the other employees started reporting symptoms. The first person was advised by her allergist to go to work wearing a respirator. Of course," he says sarcastically, "as soon as you walk into a building wearing a respirator, you're completely unnoticed by your colleagues."

Within a day the employee's union contacted the Alaska state epidemiologist, who sent in a team of industrial hygienists. "They said, 'Wait a minute, what's in this building? We don't know. Maybe there's asbestos in this building.' So they went in in full protective clothing."

That alerted the media. That evening the news featured the hygienists, in space suits, going into the building, then finally coming out to announce that there was absolutely nothing wrong. Sure, there was nothing wrong. The media decided that there was a mystery bug in the building.

"At that stage, a state epidemiologist got involved," says Hedge. "But it was a junior epidemiologist. There was so much publicity that this person became convinced there was indeed a mystery bug. He decided that the thing to do was to survey every occupant in the building and compare their responses to all the occupants in an adjacent building with a similar space layout, a similar ventilation system."

The analysis was completed quickly. There *was* a dramatic difference between reactions in the two buildings. So the only solution was to evacuate the sick building. Within a week it was empty, and it remained that way for six months. But no one ever found out what the source of the problem was.

"After a while I got involved and looked at the data they collected," Hedge goes on. "What I found was that they had made a mistake in the computer analysis. They did it so quickly that they had made a classification error. When you corrected for that, *there was no difference* between the two buildings." In other words, the whole business had been a mistake.

Hedge's conclusion? "Sick building syndrome is not a disease in the conventional sense of a disease. It's not even clear that it exists. It's a phenomenon that relates to the design of certain buildings, but we really don't know what the design elements are that affect that phenomenon. It clearly, *clearly* is related to the organizational dynamics in the building, and the psychological state of the people in the building. I suspect it relates very strongly to their beliefs about chemicals in the environment and general health." In other words, it's all in the head.

What about alternative treatments for MCS? Sauna therapy, for example? "Incredibly bizarre," says Straight. He considers evidence for any benefits from sauna therapy to be largely anecdotal, with most of the scientific studies being unconvincing, lacking controls or specific data or both.

But the skepticism directed toward these concepts and treatments is nothing compared to the scorn heaped on another linchpin of environmental medicine, provocation-neutralization therapy. Here again, the big guns — the American Medical Association, the American Academy of Allergy and Immunology, and the American College of Physicians — have come out against the procedure. "Numerous organizations have all looked at that technique and found it to be totally bogus — and I would agree," says Straight.

So does Donald Black. "There's no evidence to support it. Most mainstream allergists would say that."

These opinions are based on studies such as one conducted by University of California, San Francisco, researcher Don Jewett that appeared in 1990 in the *New England Journal of Medicine*. In an attempt to prove or disprove the validity of P/N testing, he gave eighteen patients injections of food and chemical extracts and injections of placebos and recorded their reactions to see if there was any difference. This study had a particular wrinkle, however: Jewett didn't select the patients. Rather, several clinical ecologists did. And these weren't any old patients — all of them had already reacted strongly to P/N doses and not to placebo doses. In other words, they were ringers, perfect foils to demonstrate the *validity*, not the futility, of the technique. And Jewett further bent backward to mollify environmental docs. "Before undertaking the study, we sent the protocol to both advocates and critics of provocation testing and modified it until most agreed that it was a fair and appropriate test of the method," he writes. The people would be tested with the same extracts in the same office by the same technician as before, and, if they saw something amiss, the environmental doctors could withdraw their patients.

Furthermore, the experiment would be double-blind. The person being tested wouldn't know in advance what was coming — that was a given. Now the person doing the testing wouldn't know either. There would be no possibility that a tester's body language or facial expression or any other subtle signs might give away which dose was which. This experiment, once and for all, would establish the effectiveness of P/N testing for better or for worse.

It turned out for worse. "The responses of the patients to the active and control injections were indistinguishable," writes Jewett. The symptoms generated by the extracts and placebos were identical. The provocation doses provoked nothing that placebos didn't provoke as well. So much for reproducing symptoms on the spot. Moreover, the tester gave seven of the patients neutralizing injections, and they were just as effective in relieving symptoms provoked by the placebos as they were in relieving reactions to the real things. P/N was worthless.

"We certainly did not expect the results that we obtained in these studies, since we had observed unblinded clinical testing in which active injections seemed to provoke symptoms readily," Jewett writes. The suggestion was obvious: "The symptoms were placebo responses, generated spontaneously.... We conclude that the technique as practiced works only if practiced unblinded — that is, under the influence of direct or indirect suggestion." In other words, provocation-neutralization testing is a sham.

Most mainstream physicians may be convinced, but David King isn't. A psychiatrist at the University of California, San Francisco, King has made it a point to analyze various studies of provocation-neutralization to assess their worth. He's found major limitations. Before Jewett's experiment was even published, King raised three possible concerns. The first concern gave a nod to the possibility of masking by raising the question of what the subjects of the study had been eating before the trial. If they had been avoiding the foods in question, it's possible they might have lost their prior sensitivity. Jewett's report mentioned nothing about that. The second concern was whether subtle reactions might not have been lost in the either-or conditions enforced by the trial. Some reactions simply may have been too mild to definitively place in one category or the other. Finally, King was uneasy about the size of the doses used in the trial. For a number of reasons (one being that there was less chance of a skin reaction that would compromise the double-blinding), the doses were very small. Perhaps they were too small to be effective, whereas larger doses might have provoked more reliable reactions.

King himself has reservations about the utility of P/N, but his mistrust of the methods used in the Jewett trial, as well as in others, prompts him to state that "a close examination of other frequently cited evaluation studies reveals similar flaws, making firm conclusions about provocative testing premature."

No matter their worth, none of these studies seem to faze environmental docs. For many of them, seeing is believing. They don't need sophisticated studies to tell them if their treatments work. They know they work — from experience. "In our clinic, provocation-neutralization is eighty percent effective," says Bill Rea. He and his colleagues cheerfully admit that they don't even know *how* P/N works, but that doesn't bother them either.

"Nobody knows how it works," Rea says. "It could be through the immune system, could be through the mediator systems, could be through the pharmacological systems, could be electrical. It's probably all of those, maybe things we don't understand. I really don't care. All I know is that it works."

But that's not good enough for everyone. In particular, it's not good enough for Jack Selner. That kind of attitude infuriates him. How can you prescribe a treatment that cannot be *proven* to work? That's the worst kind of charlatanism. In fact, he sees the kind of quibbling indulged in by King as symptomatic of the entire field of environmental medicine. It's a way of evading the truth.

Selner wrote a scathing review of a book about MCS that described Jewett's study and King's objections. "The secret is finally out. The tenets of clinical ecology are *not testable* within a context acceptable to ecologists," he declared. "Others should study this scientific Rubik's Cube; it appears to be a great way to perpetrate an illusion.

"This reviewer would anticipate that any results from double-blind testing carried out in an elaborately designed institutional setting will meet with the same objections from the same pseudoscientists. The testing procedures were not done long enough, or they were done too long, using not high enough, or too high, a dose under circumstances in which some other variable either *was* present or *was not* present. Thus, the intellectual merry-go-round of anecdote and fantasy will continue to be perpetuated. Unfortunately, the big losers will be the ever-increasing number of helpless and hopeless patients . . ."

In the final analysis, then, mainstream physicians feel environmental medicine is not only misguided but may be dangerous. Donald Black's opinion is characteristic. "You have to look at the weight of evidence," he says. "The way the debate is portrayed in the lay literature is that it's between people who have equally valid opinions. That's a total misconception. It's a debate among the mainstream of medicine versus a rather small but vocal group of nontraditional physicians who have not carried their part of the discussion in terms of bringing forth convincing data. If they don't have the data, why should I as a mainstream physician change my way of practicing and accommodate to views that sound to me very strange and unorthodox?"

Physicians and patients who do give it a chance are taking a huge risk. "I've seen a lot of people that I'd call pathetic," says Black. "Their lives are pathetic and in many cases ruined because of the clinical ecologists' recommendations. Once these people are taken in with this concept, and embraced by the 'chemically ill' community, it's almost like a cult."

There you have it: MCS is a cult. Cults and cultish behavior — that's an area that Herman Staudenmayer knows a lot about. "We know that social isolation is one of the primary techniques used in brainwashing, and in breaking down prisoners of war," he says. "There's extensive literature written in the early fifties on those techniques, through the Chinese in the Korean War. Some of the processes described there are *shockingly* similar to those used by clinical ecologists. At least the psychological aspects are — there are none of the physical, torturous aspects involved. The psychological techniques of brainwashing are social isolation, regimen, nonallowance of disbelief, and reinforcement of the belief. All of those are used by clinical ecologists."

"And this is a conscious strategy on their part?" I ask.

"I can't say definitively," Staudenmayer replies. "All I can do is lay out the different type of processes that have been identified in cult-type movements and in quack movements. You make the comparisons yourself."

Chapter 5

TILT!

"MCS IS HERE BECAUSE of the failure of organized medicine to resolve the issue," admits Michael Straight. "People go from doc to doc, who say, 'I don't know,' which is a perfectly honest thing to say, but it's not very satisfying. People need explanations, but instead they get labeled as crocks. So they're resentful of organized medicine. Then they find these physicians who have taken advantage of their resentment and minister to them because nobody else can — or will. They provide a support group that legitimizes the illness and labels these patients as something other than crazy.

"But these physicians tend to be not very sophisticated medically. At least judging from their reports I've seen, they have trouble spelling much less understanding complex physiology. The amount of research coming out of that community is very small and virtually worthless."

So say mainstream physicians. Environmental docs, of course, dispute the charge. When it comes to MCS, it's hard to find anyone who doesn't take sides. That's why Claudia Miller is so refreshing. A youthful forty-nine-year-old allergist-immunologist at the University of Texas Health Science Center in San Antonio, Miller has treated MCS patients and is particularly interested in the problem as a researcher. She cowrote *Chemical Exposures: Low Levels and High Stakes,* the book on chemical sensitivity that Jack Selner reviewed so angrily. In contrast to Selner's opinion — he blasted her book as distorting the problem of MCS and promoting clinical ecology — Miller sees herself as doggedly trying to walk the tightrope between the two sides. "I try to stand in the middle of all this and say, 'Let's have some rational science.' I don't attack either side. I understand the points of view on each side." Nevertheless, she's happy to be in the mainstream. "I wouldn't dare do many of the things the clinical ecologists do. Frankly, it's very dangerous. Not necessarily to the patient, but to the physician. You would be criticized, you would be attacked."

Miller may be unique among her medical colleagues in that she became involved in chemical sensitivity before she even thought of becoming a physician. For twelve years she was an industrial hygienist, first for the University of California Medical Center in San Francisco, then for the Occupational Safety and Health Administration (OSHA), and finally for the United Steelworkers Union. "I've been in mines, smelters, foundries, steel mills, and manufacturing plants of all kinds," she says. "It was a very compelling and eye-opening experience. I realize what people must do to make a living and what they are exposed to in the process."

One of the things they're exposed to is chemicals, chemicals, and more chemicals. In the mid-1970s, Miller investigated a series of unexplained illnesses at an electronics plant in Pennsylvania. Dozens of solderers, mostly women, were complaining of headaches, nausea, difficulty concentrating. Federal investigators blamed psychological causes. Miller had other ideas.

"The women were breathing a cloud of organic and inorganic chemicals from the solder fumes," she recalls. "Some of

us wondered if the cause might not be these low-level chemical exposures. Our thinking was that maybe levels that meet
OSHA standards aren't always safe for everybody." When Miller persuaded the company to install exhaust hoods to ventilate
the soldering area, the illnesses disappeared.

Experiences like that persuaded her that sensitivity to chemicals was a real and important concern, and that to deal with it
most effectively she would have to become a physician. Today
she does research in environmental and occupational health in
the University of Texas Health Science Center's Department of
Family Practice. And she finds herself one of the few mainstream physicians who is willing to take MCS seriously. As
such, she's sick and tired of the enmity between the conventional docs like her and the clinical ecologists. "The name-
calling and cross fire between the groups has been detrimental
to the patients."

That is a shame, because the groping, unsettled search for
MCS treatments simply reflects the nature of innovation and
change. "Any emerging area goes through growing pains," Miller says. "Look at the history of medicine. Leeches, bleeding,
all kinds of bizarre things happened before people found out
about the mechanisms of disease.

"MCS is at the stage where we're saying, 'There's something going on here, and this is a different process of disease, a
different mechanism from what we've seen before.' There are
lots of arguments about it, but that's typical for an emerging
area."

Yet another, surprising, reason for the lack of credence
given MCS by conventional physicians may involve their own
training. "Many physicians tend to be fairly insensitive to chemicals," Miller says. "They have to go through organic chemistry
labs, become exposed to formaldehyde in gross anatomy labs.
That kind of thing tends to weed out the chemically sensitive
people. And people who aren't real sensitive tend to be real

skeptical. Whereas people who are very sensitive, even though they don't have MCS, tend to be more understanding."

And when we talk in her office in San Antonio, Miller doesn't hesitate to needle me concerning my own role in fostering the controversy: "The media has not helped things," she says. "The sensationalizing, the exaggeration. The people who live in aluminum foil–lined rooms, on top of mountains, or isolated, like in Wimberley, make very good stories. But they're extreme. People can't identify with them. They look like they're crazy because they're living such extreme lives. Yet there are thousands of MCS patients who day to day are just barely coping, trying to work and maintain normal lives. Those people don't want anything to do with the media. So there's really a distortion."

As a result, most mainstream docs bring to MCS biased, secondhand opinions. "Many physicians have never seen a prototypical MCS patient. Or if they have, they haven't known what they were seeing. Television has colored their view."

Miller's allegiance is clearly to the patients. And she's not at all shy about criticizing her colleagues in the mainstream for their own ignorance.

An example: In September of 1995 Miller attends an MCS conference in Princeton, New Jersey, in a hotel just down the street from the university. So do I. Here environmental physicians are represented, Bill Rea and Jerry Ross among them. Here also are a few mainstream docs who treat MCS patients and some who don't. Most of the people, however, are toxicologists, laboratory researchers, academics. They've seen relatively few, if any, people with chemical sensitivity. But that doesn't stop them from making pronouncements about the problem. It sometimes seems as though the people who know the least make a point of saying the most. When it's Miller's turn to speak, she steps to the podium and asks the audience to help her with a brief survey.

"I'd like to take a little chance here and ask those of you who are either clinicians and/or researchers to stand up," she says. Most everyone of the hundred or so people in the hotel ballroom take their feet.

"If you have seen one or more patients who report being chemically sensitive, remain standing," she says. "Everyone else sit down." Perhaps half the people remain upright.

"Okay. If you've seen ten or more patients who report being chemically sensitive, remain standing. Everyone else sit down." Now there is only a handful left.

"If you've seen a hundred or more, remain standing, and the others sit down." Rea and Ross and a couple of others still stand, now conspicuously alone, looking curiously about the room.

"Okay. Thank you," Miller says. "That's a good perspective." Then, as if an afterthought, mischievously: "A thousand or more?"

Only Rea remains.

Of course, seeing a lot of patients doesn't necessarily mean that you have an answer to the problem. But it does help in trying to understand it. Which later in the conference makes a confrontation so sadly characteristic of the gulf between the sides.

Rea is the last speaker of the day. With typical brusque assurance, he offers a comprehensive plan to identify and study MCS based on his long experience in Dallas. As a backup, he's written and circulated a ninety-page discourse on the subject, complete with over 250 research references. After he speaks, members of the audience gather at the podium to voice reactions. Among them is a researcher from the Environmental Protection Agency — one of the people who quickly took their seats during Miller's survey.

"While I appreciate the fact that Dr. Rea went to the trouble to pass out his ninety-page document," the man says, sarcastically, "I don't find it very helpful, or even understandable. Besides, how is one supposed to trust Rea's work when his references aren't even from peer-reviewed journals?" In other words, not only are Rea's comments irrelevant, the questionable credentials for his references undermine his ideas. In this case, guilt by *lack* of association.

Afterward, as people file out to dinner, Rea confronts the man. "What do you mean 'not peer-reviewed'?"

The EPA researcher is startled, and a little embarrassed. "What I mean is that they're obscure and hard to find. A lot of them are in German journals."

"That's different," says Rea. "Those kinds of accusations are thrown at me all the time. There's a big difference between saying they're not peer-reviewed and that they're hard to find. That's a problem with your medical library, not with me, okay?"

The man sheepishly backs down.

No matter. His point was all too clear and, as Rea was unable to rebut his remarks during the meeting, all too effective. Most people in the mainstream consider the science and treatment methods coming out of the ecologist camp suspect — *even if they know absolutely nothing about them.* And one of the reasons for that skepticism concerns the journals, peer-reviewed or not, where papers from environmental medicine practitioners often show up. *Clinical Ecology,* for example. It is peer-reviewed, but it may not have the same rigorous standards as more prominent journals. Rarely do you find environmental medicine papers in prominent establishment periodicals such as the *New England Journal of Medicine,* or the *Journal of the American Medical Association.* Why is that?

Miller offers an answer. "When you look at a lot of things Rea and other ecologists have written, they don't meet the standards of the *New England Journal* or any other major journal," she says. "People criticize them for that. Yet these people did not go into practice to be researchers — and perhaps some of them need help in designing studies. Somebody needs to pick up the ball and do these studies right. Instead, the ecologists get blamed for not proving their things the way they need to prove them."

But if not everything coming out of environmental medicine rates exposure in the best mainstream journals, you'd think *something* would. In at least some cases, suggests Miller, the exclusion is due to simple bias.

"When it comes to MCS, it's more difficult to have anything published in mainstream journals, whereas something in another field with the same level of scientific merit might be," she says. "The standards for MCS papers are much more exacting, scrutiny is much more intense, because many scientists don't believe it exists."

"There is real bias, there surely is," agrees Jerry Ross. "I used to think it was paranoid to think that, but there *is* bias. The *New England Journal* had an article some years ago — the Jewett article [which concluded that provocation-neutralization testing was worthless; see chapter 4]. After it was published, a consortium of people wrote in, citing its obvious flaws. Of course there was no way the journal would publish an article in response.

"Another situation: one of our colleagues — not in environmental medicine, but an ordinary academic physician in another discipline — put together an article and cited Bill Rea's work. He submitted it to a well-known journal, one of the top ones. And he got a call from somebody in editorial who said, 'If you expect to publish in this journal you will *not* cite any work by Bill Rea.'"

"How does it feel to be belittled like that?" I ask.

"It does bother a person," Ross replies. "I have to battle against the us-versus-them kind of attitude. There are a lot of very well meaning people out there who are not informed.

They parrot what they are taught by the system in which they receive their information, without much critical thought."

Characteristically, Rea takes a tougher line: "I don't look at this as sides, okay? Selner's bunch? We don't even respond to them. I'm used to being called a quack." He gives a belly laugh. "They're empty words. Nonsense. Doesn't bother me.

"You have to remember that probably sixty, eighty percent of medicine is ignorant about all this. They just don't know. The horrible part is it becomes the patients' problem. But that's not our fault. We're pedaling as fast as we can."

Doris Rapp didn't attend the Princeton conference. But her experience has been much like Rea's — despite her mainstream credentials.

"I practiced straight pediatric allergy medicine until 1975," she says. "Then I went to a food-allergy meeting in Miami. I went to hear traditional allergists, but some of these quacks were on the program. The traditional allergists were doing things just the way I was. But these other guys said that dust and molds and pollen could cause behavior and learning problems. They could cause bellyaches and bed-wetting and all these other things. I said, 'Come on, you've got to be kidding.'

"I sat in the first row, trying to figure it out. And the thing that impressed me was that while the traditional doctors like me were using lots of medicines and everything else, these quacky doctors rarely had someone on steroids and didn't have to order much medicine. I said, 'They're lying.'

"After that meeting I decided to check on these guys. So I went to a doc who's doing this in Texas. She was seeing a patient, and I said, 'There's a new drug that will be perfect until you get this patient treated.' She said, 'Okay, let's try it.' It took her *ten minutes* to find a prescription pad in her office. That was a revelation.

"I asked for a demonstration of provocation-neutralization. She brought in some patients, and she turned them on and off just like I'm doing now all the time. I looked at it and said, 'This is a setup. You're fooling me.'

"Then I went to another environmental doctor, in Mobile, Alabama. At the end of three days I came back to my husband and said, 'The guy's so clever he's duped me.' He was making people wheeze, causing hyperactivity, making their noses run, doubling them up with bellyaches, then making it all stop.

"So I tried it myself. The first patient I tried, I doubled her up and her belly swelled way up. I thought she was fooling. I gave her the wrong neutralization dilutions, because I didn't believe a weak dilution could do anything. I did everything wrong, and she got progressively worse. Finally I did just what I had been told at that meeting, and I stopped the reaction."

With that, Rapp started using these techniques in her own practice. And she determined to convince her colleagues that the methods worked. "I thought all I had to do was double-blinded studies and they'd listen. So I did them. But when I tried to publish them, they were accepted into journals of learning disabilities, not in the medical journals. Finally I got an article published in the *Medical Journal of Australia*. Well, who the hell reads the *Medical Journal of Australia?*"

Rapp suddenly found herself on the other side of the tracks. "I was ostracized," she says. "I'd go to a medical meeting, and my friends for years would say, 'Oh, Doris, it's so nice to see you.' Then they'd turn around and go the other way. No one would sit with me at the table. At one point the powers that be told me I couldn't use my clinical title on anything I published unless it was approved by the head of pediatrics at the hospital. I was told I couldn't work in the allergy clinic in the hospital anymore.

"I was very embarrassed. I can remember one meeting when I saw one of my mentors in environmental medicine, and I turned the other way for fear somebody would know I knew him. I'm still ashamed. I was afraid to have my name put in the list of environmental medical doctors.

"I would still go home and say, 'Doris, are you deceiving yourself? Did you really see that kid get better? Do you think all this really helps?' Then the next morning I'd go into the office and a mother would throw her arms around me and say, 'I just can't thank you enough. My child hasn't wheezed for three months. My child doesn't bite me in the morning when he gets out of bed.'

"So I said, 'Doris, you have to do more research. You have to document what you see.' I spent a fortune on videos. You want to see that dust causes hyperactivity in a three-year-old? I've got a video of it. You tell me what you want, I've got videos of all of it.

"But people said that the kids were acting, because they were older kids. So I got younger kids. Then they said that the kids were tired or irritable because they needed a nap. You can't win.

"Finally I said, 'Doris, forget it. You're a real schnook. They are never going to believe you. You're a clinician, someone who sees patients. You're not an academician, you can't do research on a big scale.' But I say, academics ought to listen to what we're saying. If they can't help patients, why won't they at least let us try to help?"

Claudia Miller agrees. What this turmoil should not do, she insists, is get in the way of prevention — even if disease theories are not backed by experimental proof. The history of medicine is replete with instances in which physicians acted first and looked for proof later. As a prime example, Miller points to John Snow and his fight against cholera.

It's a famous story in medical circles. In the middle of the nineteenth century, a devastating epidemic of cholera descended upon England. Snow, a London anesthesiologist who lived in the Soho district of the city, took it upon himself to look into a local outbreak that had claimed over five hundred lives in just ten days. The prevailing theory at the time was that cholera was caused by miasmas, foul emanations wafting through the air. Snow suspected otherwise. He noticed that in the heart of the neighborhood, at the intersection of Broad and Cambridge streets, was a water pump used by virtually everyone. Rather than these vague miasmas, might not the disease be the result of something in the water? Snow decided to find out.

Snow drew a map of the area, marking deaths with tiny coffins. He found that they clustered in the streets surrounding the pump like iron filings around a magnet. The circumstantial evidence was compelling. But then Snow was confronted with exceptions, among them the puzzling circumstance that none of the seventy employees at a nearby Broad Street brewery had come down with the disease. If the water was at fault, surely some of them should be dead.

Snow interviewed the brew master, and soon the solution to the puzzle became clear: the men drank only beer. They had never once used the pump. That was why, in the midst of death, they had survived. The exception had proved the rule. Snow convinced the city officials to remove the handle from the Broad Street pump, and the epidemic subsided.

The point is, Snow didn't know what caused cholera. He simply did something about it. "Robert Koch came along thirty years after the cholera epidemic in London, and he identified the bacterium, and everything fell into place," says Miller. "If we had a marker for chemical sensitivity as clear as the bacterium that Koch saw, all the arguments would end overnight. But now we're in this theorizing stage, which is a very difficult time, one in which a lot of people are uncomfortable. Physicians don't like uncertainty. But that's what we have to tolerate now.

"We're at the stage where there are things we can do to intervene well before we know the mechanism. You have to base logical intervention on observation when you don't know the mechanism."

(A sidebar: A couple of Question-and-Answer sessions during the Princeton conference were opened to the community. Suddenly these physicians and researchers, many of whom had flunked Claudia Miller's stand-up test — and few of whom showed up to meet the public — found themselves face to face with actual MCS sufferers. During discussions, the name of John Snow came up.

"Why can't you be like Snow and try to do something about the problem even before you understand the cause?" came the question.

"John Snow died forgotten and penniless," was one doc's answer. It's easy to talk about going against convention — it's harder to actually do it. You run the risk of ending up like John Snow.

Or, he might have said, "like Bill Rea," whose very name as a reference is enough to prevent an article from being published in a mainstream medical journal.)

San Francisco immunologist Al Levin (pronounced Le-*vin*) considers the whole brouhaha inexpressibly stupid. "My foundation was immunology. But I've worked with clinical ecologists. That the so-called traditional allergists think that they have good science and that the so-called clinical ecologists have bad science is ridiculous. It's like the left-handed surgeon arguing with the right-handed surgeon about how to take out a gall bladder. They're doing the same thing in a little different way. But the differences are meaningless. There are good medical people on both sides — absolutely, no problem! They complement each other."

It's a minority view of the situation, but Levin offers minority — and provocative — views on just about everything.
"Al Levin is a kamikaze," says Rea.

Levin laughs. "That's right. Except I'm still alive."

Which is saying a great deal. Small and slim, with close-
cropped dark hair and an angular face, Levin today is an ani-
mated, feisty fifty-nine-year-old. In 1966, recently graduated
from the University of Illinois medical school, he found himself drafted out of an internship at Harvard and Children's Hospital in Boston to train as a flight surgeon for the navy. In no
time at all he was transported to Vietnam.

Once there, it wasn't long before Levin became involved
in some of the darker episodes in the American entanglement
in Southeast Asia. For example, he found himself smack-dab in
the middle of the drug trade. For four months he flew air support for a covert CIA-sponsored effort to convey heroin out
of Burma and Laos and into the United States. The transport
planes, flown by military personnel, went by many names. "Air
America, Evergreen Airlines, Southern Air Transport — big
white airplanes with any name you wanted on them," he recalls. "We used to call the operation Air No Name. And the
pilots — one day they'd be colonels in the marine corps, next
day captains in the army, next day Bechtel engineers. They had
a dozen different ID cards. Get 'em drunk and they wouldn't
know who they were."

He also was part of clandestine assassination teams. "The
theory was that you destroy the family of the village chieftain,
but you don't destroy him. He then loses confidence and loses
control of the village. That's what we did — we'd go in and kill
women and children. Some of the guys were special forces,
some were SEALs, some were civilians, and some were like
me, active-duty military. It was very well run. I have a great
deal of respect for how the CIA runs their operations."

Shaken by these and other misadventures ("For thirteen
months I ate, slept, and drank Agent Orange," he says. "I'm just

waiting for cancer") and bearing a chestful of medals and commendations, including the Silver Star, Levin arrived in San Francisco late in 1969, disillusioned, angry, and determined to resurrect a medical career that might allow him to save rather than kill people for a change. It wasn't long before he ran into more controversy — and MCS.

"The reason I got interested in this whole area was that in 1974 I met a clinical ecologist named Phyllis Saifer. I thought she was a quack, delightful but nuts. She told me about all these people who were allergic to perfumes and all these other things. She said, 'What do I do to find out if their immune systems are damaged?' I told her, 'Check their B and T cells.' Then I kind of forgot about it."

As an immunologist, Levin knew better than most that B and T cells, vital disease-fighting white blood cells, offered a window into the immune system. If B- and T-cell levels were normal, odds were the immune system was functioning well. If not, it might be depressed. (For example, measuring T-cell levels is a prime way of detecting AIDS. The fewer the T cells, the more likely that disease is on its way.) As he had become a director of an immunology lab, as well as a staff physician at the University of California, San Francisco, Levin was well set up to ascertain those levels. The technicians in his lab routinely evaluated blood samples from various docs all over the Bay area. Then one day something happened that was not routine.

"A technician ran into my office and said, 'There's something wrong with our assays,'" Levin recalls.

"'Why?' I said.

"'Because everybody's got low T cells.'

"I walked out to the lab bench and checked things out. I discovered that all these blood samples were from Saifer's patients. At that point the only people who we knew had T-cell problems were cancer patients. I thought, 'She's a closet oncologist. She's seeing cancer patients.'

"So, with her permission I called the patients into the office and interviewed them. They all described the same symptoms, MCS symptoms. The interesting thing was, I would always ask my cancer patients, 'What were you like before you developed the disease?' And they almost always described these same symptoms.

"So I went back to Phyllis and said, 'Look, these people have cancer.' And as we expanded looking at these people, we found that it's not only cancer, it's autoimmune disease, thyroid disease, in some cases multiple sclerosis. If you talk to anybody who takes care of lupus patients, they'll tell you that these people have the same symptoms. It all made sense. It was perfectly logical that what we were looking at was immune disregulation that presented itself as a disease process down the line."

For Levin, then, MCS is a harbinger of something else, something more dire — cancer, lupus, MS, even diabetes. He has now followed MCS patients over two decades, to find that many end up with these very diseases. "We are now claiming that if you have MCS, you have a fifty-one percent chance of getting either cancer or autoimmune disease," he says. "That's for the people who just don't get better. If they're appropriately treated, they may not develop these diseases, or their disease may not be as severe as otherwise." He suspects that people who suffer MCS have a genetic propensity to suffer serious disease triggered by exposure to the environment. And the first symptom of that triggering is MCS.

Levin thinks that four mechanisms are primarily involved in the disorder. It may be that toxic chemicals induce white blood cells to commit suicide — a process called apoptosis. And, as AIDS makes all too clear, loss of white blood cells depletes the immune system. Another possible mechanism involves the effect of chemicals on the thymus gland. The thymus functions as a halfway house for T cells — they pass through the gland for processing and maturation. Levin suspects that a chemically damaged thymus might pass defective cells into the body — in particular, cells that might attack the body's own tissue, causing autoimmune disease. It also may be that toxic chemicals damage DNA enzymes, causing cells to die or perhaps even produce cancer-causing genes, or oncogenes. And finally, chemicals might trigger already existing, but quiescent, oncogenes, causing the gradual development of cancer down the line.

For Levin, then, far from not displaying any telltale laboratory signs, MCS offers clear and consistent markers. They're the same ones that are present in cancer and autoimmune disease, for which MCS is prelude. "These people have immune disorders," he says. "The evidence is quite uniform."

Chief among the signs of these disorders is the ratio between levels of two specific kinds of T cells: helper T cells and suppressor T cells. The roles these cells play in maintaining health is crucial. Helper T cells, so-called CD4+ cells, regulate the immune system. In the event of an onslaught by foreign invaders such as viruses and bacteria, they cause B cells to spring into action and produce antibodies, and they direct other kinds of T cells to engage the enemies directly and kill them. Without helper T cells, there wouldn't be much of an immune response at all. But once these cells repel the invasion, they must be stopped and sent home, or the armada of disease-fighting cells, with nothing left to fight, might turn on the body itself and cause autoimmune disease. That's the role of suppressor T cells, CD8+ cells, which suppress the action of the attack cells and shut down the immune response. To work efficiently, then, the immune system must have a healthy ratio between these two kinds of T cells, about two helper cells to every one suppressor cell. In most people, that's just what the ratio is.

Not in MCS sufferers, however. Here, Levin finds, the ratio between helper Ts and suppressor Ts is unstable and erratic. In fact, in people exposed to toxic levels of formaldehyde, pesticides, and herbicides, suppressor cells become predominant. That's no good. Too many suppressor cells may make for a chronically suppressed immune system. "Recovery from the syndrome is marked by a reduction of suppressor T cells and a normalization of the ratio between helpers and suppressors," Levin says.

In treating MCS sufferers, then, he tries to restore that healthy balance. Avoidance is the most important tack Levin recommends, but he also employs a variety of other treatments. Two of these, both controversial, are intravenous doses of gamma globulin and transfer factor, blood products that provide antibody and T-cell reinforcements. For most people, Levin claims, the treatment works. "The overwhelming majority of people, eighty-five percent of them, get over MCS," he says. "The hardcore people, the fifteen percent, they're the ones who come down with something later. They have a forerunner illness."

In this light, the importance of doing something about MCS, and doing it early on, skyrockets. "The scientific value of identifying this disease process is enormous," Levin says. "If you can treat cancer or autoimmune disease long before it becomes clinically significant, you can do a whole lot to turn it around. And you can study the basic biochemistry of the disease. That's finally happening now. But it has taken a long time and has been real bloody, a real bitter battle."

Rebecca Bascom, a no-nonsense pulmonary specialist at the University of Maryland School of Medicine in Baltimore who sees MCS patients, suggests a more homely scenario. She suspects that MCS involves a important nerve located in the front part of the head — the trigeminal nerve — and a naturally occurring protein called substance P.

The trigeminal nerve relays to the brain information from the front part of the head, including the nose and mouth, about temperature, pain, and touch. It's known that certain chemical irritants can inflame the fibers in the nerve, causing the release of a pain-provoking small protein, or peptide, called substance P. Substance P does more than simply cause pain; it also induces mast cells to jettison their cargo of potent granules. That means an allergic reaction — even more inflammation, itching, and other unpleasantness.

For Bascom, then, odds are that MCS is at heart a respiratory disorder. "The basic idea is that in order for the body to respond to an irritant, there has to be a pathway from sensing it to responding to it," she says. "In most of the people I see, the route of exposure is through inhalation. The first point of contact of the material coming in is with the respiratory tissue and the mucosal surface."

Once there, enzymes in the inhaled chemicals may break down the tissue or the fluid that bathes it. As a result, the tissue may produce substances that stimulate underlying nerve fibers, or the chemicals themselves may make contact with the nerves. And as a result of that stimulation, the fibers may produce substance P as well as other nerve-stimulating materials. "They can be released locally and cause local effects. And they can also be released centrally and stimulate systemic reflexes," Bascom says.

She has an ally in Bill Meggs. A physician-toxicologist who divides his time between the Department of Emergency Medicine at East Carolina University in Greenville, North Carolina, and the New York City Poison Center in Manhattan, Meggs also points to substance P and respiratory problems as a likely instigator of MCS. He offers a scenario explaining how a local, upper-airway disorder can result in whole-body symptoms, even neurological and psychological symptoms. There's precedent for that kind of dissemination right under our noses: common allergies. "Patients with allergies have symptoms at sites other than the site of inoculation with an allergen," he says in his soft Carolina drawl. For example, hay fever can do more than just make you sneeze. It can also cause headaches and fatigue. "And the mechanism may be identical in patients with chemical sensitivity."

In Meggs's view, the process develops this way. Inhaling a chemical produces inflammation in the upper airway, which itself produces local allergy-like irritation. In turn, the inflamed tissue produces proteins that attract immune-system defenders, such as white blood cells. Upon subsequent chemical exposures, those white blood cells release other immune-system agents, including hormones that have an effect on the central nervous system. Thus the beginning of whole-body symptoms — nausea, muscle pains, fatigue. And the process may also activate stress pathways in the body that produce the psychological manifestations of MCS. But it all starts with a sniff of a toxic chemical.

With that, Bascom can agree. But she won't endorse the rest. In fact, she won't even go along with the idea of inflammation being one of the consequences of chemical exposure. "We don't know if there is inflammation. That's why this is just a hypothesis. A reasonable hypothesis, but it hasn't been tested." To do so would require taking a biopsy of the tissues involved and comparing them to those of people with similar problems but no exposure to chemical irritants. Or, to confirm the existence of these sensitivities if not their cause, it might be possible to do experiments similar to one Bascom and her colleagues performed in 1990 to measure reactions to cigarette smoke. They exposed ten people with a history of smoke sensitivity and eleven "normal" people to fifteen minutes of smoke followed by fifteen minutes of clean air ("We chose a relatively high concentration of sidestream tobacco smoke, similar to that measured in bars or taverns," she explains) and then measured their reactions. The smoke-sensitive people, but not the "normals," experienced increased nasal congestion, headache, chest discomfort or tightness, and cough. They also were afflicted with runny noses and throat and nose irritations more than the other group. But all that without the irritating presence of histamine, suggesting that neither mast cells nor IgE were involved in the reaction. The irritation was real, all right, but whatever was happening was outside the conventional boundaries of allergy.

Until there's more evidence concerning MCS, then, Bascom refuses to commit herself. The problem is simply too hard to pin down.

In collaboration with University of Arizona psychiatrist Iris Bell, Claudia Miller herself has come up with an intriguing hypothesis that may serve to tie together those who feel that MCS is all in the head and those who contend that it is a physiological illness (especially those, like Bascom and Meggs, who emphasize the possible involvement of upper-airway disorders).

Bell is the researcher who conducted the chemical sensitivity surveys of college students and elderly people that suggested at least 15 percent of the population is sensitive to a variety of chemicals. The focus of her and Miller's approach is the limbic portion of the brain, a network of small structures including the hippocampus, hypothalamus, and amygdala that form a ring (or "limbus") surrounding the brain stem. It is this area of the brain that affects our mood and emotions, that is essential for forming new memories, and that influences hormone production and the function of the involuntary nervous system. Fear, rage, aggression, pleasure, sex drive, and reproductive cycles — all these are generated by the limbic system. And all these are involved in the kinds of behaviors that go awry in MCS. It just so happens that the limbic system is the region of the brain most closely connected to the environment — through our sense of smell. Nerves that convey odors begin in the nose and end up in a small area of the brain called the olfactory bulb, which resides right next door to the limbic system. Whatever the nose smells makes a beeline to the brain via this nonstop superhighway.

Therefore, Bell and Miller suggest, toxic environmental chemicals may gain direct access to the nervous system along this route, kindle, or sensitize, it, and thus cause the disturbing spectrum of symptoms characteristic of chemical sensitivity. "This hypothesis fits a lot of the clinical observations on chemical sensitivity," says Miller. "Memory difficulties, concentration difficulties, mood changes — like walking through the detergent aisle of the grocery store and suddenly feeling angry at people, wanting to run them over with your grocery cart. That kind of response is very limbic. Neuroanatomically, this is a logical location for what's going on."

Experiments with animals are giving the theory some credence. For example, a University of Washington researcher named Barbara Sorg is exposing rodents to formaldehyde, then giving them a dose of cocaine. What she's found is that the prior exposure to formaldehyde increases the animals' sensitivity to the cocaine, a phenomenon similar to that in MCS, where exposure to a chemical seems to increase sensitization to a variety of unrelated compounds. And the seat of the sensitization is the limbic area.

In Sweden, researchers exposed animals to low concentrations of toluene, a common solvent, for about a month, after which the animals' behavior changed. They became sensitized to the toluene — again, a limbic phenomenon.

Lisa Morrow of the University of Pittsburgh is doing limbic-area research with people. She has found that workers who have been exposed to solvents are unable to slow their heart rate and reduce the size of their pupils under stressful conditions. It's as if their flight-or-fight nervous system has been activated and can't shut down, whereas people who haven't been exposed to solvents can relax more readily. "These guys were on maximum alert," says Bell. "There's potential limbic involvement in that."

Bell herself is giving Arizona University students low-level exposures to solvents, perfume, and alcohol, then measuring the response in their brains. "It's just little bottles under the nose. While they're sniffing we're looking at brain wave responses," she says. "We're still analyzing the data. It looks promising, but the process is much more complex than I hoped."

But if the limbic-kindling theory may help to explain the neurological symptoms associated with MCS, it fails to address many of the others. What about skin rashes? Nothing neurological about that. And what about patients with joint pain? Says Bill Rea (and his comment may also apply to Bascom's and Meggs's theories), "I think the theory is fine for the brain, but it doesn't have anything to do with the whole gamut of chemical sensitivity. For example, it doesn't answer the rheumatoid arthritic patients, who don't have brain dysfunction. It's not the answer to the whole picture."

And Herman Staudenmayer isn't going to budge. "My contention would be that all the explanations offered to explain the symptomatology could equally be explained by psychological effects effecting the same mechanisms in the limbic system through well-understood processes," he says. "If you look at the pyschophysiology of the human stress response, you can explain the symptomatology without postulating *any* toxicological explanation."

Nevertheless, at least with respect to some of the miseries of MCS, the warring camps might have a reason to wed. If the neurological symptoms of MCS are generated in the limbic system of the brain, the notion that the problem is all in the head — or at least *begins* in the head — is right on. And if limbic disruptions are triggered by chemical odors, the idea that MCS is an illness caused by environmental offenders is similarly on the mark. Bell and Miller are offering a bridge to span the gulf.

In fact, Bell sees merit in Selner and Staudenmayer's contention that childhood sexual abuse is the cause of MCS. "It seems plausible," she says. "Some of my research is somewhat consistent with that. But my interpretation is very different."

For example, questionnaires Bell has given her research subjects reveal that childhood stress is more prevalent in them than in normal controls. "We have at least two studies, one on MCS and one on the elderly in the community, showing evidence of increased stressfulness in early life. We did not specifically ask about childhood abuse, but we can say that we have evidence of higher stress earlier in the lives of people who say they're chemically sensitive."

Having given that nod to the work of Selner and Staudenmayer, however, Bell begs to differ. "There's a lot of evidence in basic neuroscience right now that early life stress changes the way the brain and stress response system work in very profound ways," she says. "My interpretation of our findings would be that there was a persistent change in the brain and stress response system that might have been the result of childhood abuse but is currently manifested by genuine reactivity to chemicals."

If so, are these physical changes reversible through psychotherapy, as Selner and Staudenmayer claim? "Probably not," Bell says. "Once you've activated those changes, it's very difficult to reverse them. Psychotherapy, even relaxation and meditation, are very beneficial for some of the medical conditions that MCS patients have. But they're not the cure-all for them. If somebody has psychotherapy that assists her in dampening how she reacts to stress, that can be very beneficial. Do I think it'll take away the vulnerability? No.

"I'm very concerned about the patients who may say, 'Now my MCS is gone!' Because I think they may be at risk for much more serious things down the road."

Miller agrees that limbic kindling might offer only a partial resolution of the mystery of MCS. "Limbic kindling could explain some of the brain-centered stuff," she says. "But I have trouble when I get to things like food intolerances and gastrointestinal problems and skin responses. I don't think the theory applies to everything."

Another theory might come closer. It specifically involves the way nerves fire the brain. Nerve cells in the brain are called neurons, and neurons are cells like no other. With pyramid-shaped bodies and thin tendrils called axons that extend many times the length of the cell bodies, they resemble long-legged spiders. It's along these axons that neurons generate electrical charges that trigger the release of chemical messengers called neurotransmitters. These neurotransmitters travel across minute gaps called synapses to receptors in neighboring neurons, where they spark similar electrical impulses, thereby causing the lightning storms in the brain that we experience as thought and sensation.

One of the primary neurotransmitters is a chemical called acetylcholine. The process of neurons sending acetylcholine to receptors in neurons next door is referred to as the cholinergic pathway. And here's where things get interesting. One of the functions of acetylcholine is to dampen down behavior. "There's evidence that in depressed individuals the cholinergic pathways are overactive — meaning that they have more receptors to receive acetylcholine," says pharmacologist David Overstreet of the University of North Carolina. In an attempt to pin down the mechanism involved in MCS, Overstreet is working with Miller to explore an animal model — in this case rats — for the malady. Overstreet has bred a strain of depressed rats.

That is, under certain circumstances the rats are depressed. And those circumstances mirror the chemical exposures of MCS sufferers. The similarity prompts Overstreet and Miller to suspect that MCS may involve a disruption of normal cholinergic processes in the brain. This is how their investigation has proceeded:

In the beginning, Overstreet exposed his rats to an organophosphate, a chemical contained in many commonly used
pesticides (the chemical in the rose powder that induced the
Kiessigs' woes). It had a dramatic effect on the rats — it made
them depressed. And how, you may ask, does a depressed rat
behave?

"Their sleep patterns are like those we see in depressed
people — they have elevated REM sleep," says Overstreet. "If
you look at their general activity, they're a little slower. And if
you put them under stress by giving them an electrical shock
in the foot, they become very inactive. They just sit around.
They have lower body weight, and their appetite is reduced.
That's also a problem for people who are depressed."

Overstreet separated out and bred the rats who were sensitive to organophosphates. After a while he had a whole colony
of them. "Those animals who responded in a dramatic way
were bred together; those animals who didn't show much response were bred together. We eventually developed two different strains with no overlap in their response to that particular chemical."

Now he could experiment with the rats, test them with different chemicals, investigate the physical mechanisms behind
their responses. "We began to find that they were hyperrespon-
sive to a number of other compounds," he says. "Like alcohol
and nicotine, which have also been reported to affect people
with MCS."

And, when he did brain biopsies of the depressed strain of
rats, Overstreet found that they differed from the normal rats
in one striking feature: they had many more receptors for acetylcholine. "So in rats, and people, if you have a subgroup who
have too many receptors for their own good, when acetylcholine is released, they'll get an abnormal response instead of
a normal response. Too much acetylcholine and you become
depressed, because acetylcholine is involved in behavioral in-
hibition."

Overstreet is now trying to generate funding for more experiments, experiments that might show if other neurotransmitters and other pathways in the brain are involved in MCS-like reactions. For example, if the neurotransmitter serotonin is involved — and there are indications in Overstreet's rats that it might be — a powerful avenue of treatment may be opened up. The drug Prozac acts on the serotonin pathway. And it may be that secondary pathways, set in motion by both acetylcholine and serotonin, may contribute to the problem. "MCS may be more than one biochemical condition that gives rise to the same symptoms," says Overstreet.

In any case, the promise of an animal model for MCS is encouraging. Investigations of disease move much more quickly when animals are available for experimentation. And in this case, it may be possible to perform similar experiments in humans — for example, by measuring the presence of acetylcholine receptors in white blood cells or platelets rather than having to invade the brain. The possibilities are exciting. But at present that's all they are — possibilities.

The sum of all these attempts at explaining MCS makes Miller suspect that MCS may represent a brand-new disease. Or, more precisely, a brand-new category of diseases. "Because there's no consensus on a definition of MCS, some think that MCS does not exist," she explains. "On the other hand, the reason there's no consensus could be that MCS is not a *single* syndrome, but a *collection* of syndromes that share the same general mechanism, much as cholera, influenza, and Rocky Mountain spotted fever share the same general mechanism — in this case, infectious disease."

Consider infectious disease. It's hardly been a hundred years since the germ theory of disease became medical gospel rather than upstart heresy. As a dramatic example of the way medicine was practiced pre-Pasteur, Koch, and Lister, Miller likes to point out how disease was approached in the Civil War, the world's last major conflict fought without the knowledge of infectious disease.

"Two-thirds of the deaths among soldiers during the Civil War were caused by infections, most frequently wound infections and epidemics," Miller says. Rather than basing a diagnosis on a combination of symptoms and laboratory identification of a disease agent, as physicians would today with AIDS, say, in which the clincher is provided by a blood test to detect the presence of HIV, Civil War physicians knew nothing of microbes and had to rely on symptoms alone. For example, they divided fever maladies into three categories: remittent, intermittent, and relapsing. The remittent category suggested typhoid; intermittent and relapsing pointed toward malaria. These were diseases physicians knew, but undiagnosable maladies such as typhus, TB, pneumonia, and leptospirosis — infectious diseases all — were undoubtedly present in the mix. Infectious diarrheas were a constant scourge.

"Could we be at the Civil War stage in our understanding of MCS?" asks Miller. Just as the comprehensive concept of infectious disease displaced the arcane Civil War categories, might multiple chemical sensitivity serve as a comparable umbrella for a comparable variety of problems? Just as infectious disease includes ailments that have little in common except the fact that they're caused by microbes, might MCS similarly include maladies that have nothing in common except the fact that they're caused by chemicals?

It is a provocative notion. Especially so because a comparison of MCS and infectious disease, as well as MCS and immune disease, the category that includes traditional allergy, reveals more similarities than discrepancies. For example, many of the symptoms in each category are virtually identical to the others. Fatigue, rash, headache, shortness of breath, diarrhea, general malaise — these are characteristic of infectious disease, immune disease, as well as MCS. The exposure routes of all three categories are identical: inhalation, ingestion, injection, skin/mucous membrane content. All three can affect any organ in the body, and several organs at once. And, so Miller's theory goes, all three are caused by specific, identifiable agents. Microbes in the case of infectious disease; pollen, mold, house dust mites, animal dander, foods, and drugs in immune disease; and pesticides, solvents, combustion products, drugs, and implants for MCS.

Besides offering an apt comparison, infectious disease provides a model for testing for MCS. One of the reasons infectious disease theory became established so solidly was that there arose an approach for pinning down the offending microbes. It was badly needed. During the "bacteriomania" following the widespread adoption of the germ theory of disease in the late nineteenth century, overly enthusiastic researchers claimed to have found the microbes for a variety of diseases, then were forced to retract their "discoveries" when it became clear they had found nothing. For example, researchers claimed to have found the cause of yellow fever, a viral disease, years before viruses were even discovered. To try to put a stop to the chaos, Robert Koch came up with a set of rules to verify the cause of disease. The rules are famous in medical science as Koch's Postulates.

1. The microbe must be present in every case of the disease.
2. You must be able to isolate and cultivate it in the laboratory.
3. Introducing the cultivated microbe into a healthy animal must cause the same disease.
4. You must be able to recover the microbe from the animal and cultivate it again in the lab.

Failing any of these stipulations, a disease could not be said to be caused by a microbe. The postulates were, and are, an effective way to safeguard against false claims.

Miller suggests an analogous set of conditions for MCS. Let's call them Miller's Postulates.

1. When a patient avoids all inciting chemicals, foods, and drugs (as in an ECU), symptoms disappear.
2. When any one of the same chemical, food, or drug is reintroduced to the patient, certain symptoms occur.
3. When the patient once more avoids all incitants, symptoms again disappear.
4. Upon reexposure to the same incitant no sooner than four to seven days later, the same symptoms occur again.

Why the stipulation of four to seven days between exposures? Because it takes that long for a patient to de-mask, de-adapt. And unless you can get rid of the misleading effects of masking, these tests are useless. Says Miller, "It's the equivalent of taking a ten-cup-a-day coffee drinker, giving him another cup, and asking if he gets a headache — it doesn't work."

As far as she's concerned, the importance of masking simply can't be overemphasized. It is masking that confuses physicians when they encounter MCS sufferers; it is masking that confuses the people themselves. Understanding masking is crucial to understanding MCS. "Masking is the single issue that divides the people who think something is going on with MCS and the people who don't," Miller says.

Masking is tricky. As you become used to repeated exposures to incitants, your reactions to them may change. "If you're using alcohol, tobacco, caffeine, the acute symptoms from your first exposure become more chronic as you reexpose yourself," says Miller. "If you work in a sick building, you tend to be worse on Mondays, and over the week you acclimatize." Then, after a weekend away, the reaction may be strong again the following Monday.

When people are sensitive to a number of different things

at the same time — the particular curse of multiple chemical sensitivity — the effects of those sensitivities overlap, further confusing the picture. "You've got to get rid of all this background noise before you can test patients," Miller says. "If you don't, they may have so much noise going on that they can't discern any specific cause-and-effect relationships."

In fact, many MCS patients say that at first they had no idea chemical exposures had anything to do with their problems. It wasn't until, perhaps by accident, they avoided enough offending chemicals that they noticed feeling better. Then, when they encountered them again, their symptoms returned. It's the process of avoidance and reexposure that sheds light on which chemicals trigger which symptoms.

Masking also plays a crucial role in Miller's theory of the process involved in the onset of MCS. She likens the process to an iceberg, most of which is under water. It's that tiny portion above water — the symptoms of the disease — that doctors see. And it's that same tiny portion upon which they must base their diagnosis. But masking may have distorted those symptoms. So, like an ocean liner lost in fog, physicians run into this iceberg of symptoms not knowing if what they see can be trusted. (It's a hazardous encounter for patients, as well. For even if they find doctors who know something about MCS, or are willing to entertain the possibility that it's a real problem, the docs may not know enough to consider the likelihood of masking. And, even if they do, how are they going to get rid of it without an ECU? MCS presents difficulties on almost every level.)

For Miller, then, the disease process has two stages. First is the initial exposure to an incitant. The exposure may be memorable, as in the Kiessigs' encounter with plant pesticide, the Pitmans' move to their chemically saturated new house and neighborhood, or Helen Keplinger's breathing the contaminated air in her EPA office. Or it may happen undetected over time. No matter. The effect is the same.

"You must be susceptible," says Miller. "Not everyone develops this illness." And for those who are susceptible, the central mystery of MCS takes place. "These people seem to lose tolerance to things they formerly tolerated very well and that most of us tolerate on a daily basis," says Miller.

Loss of tolerance — that's stage number one. The next stage involves triggering of the symptoms once again, this time by low-level exposures. "Subsequently, after these people have lost tolerance, and they encounter low-level exposures to food, chemicals, drugs, alcohol, and the like, the symptoms are triggered again."

All this happens below the waves — which, in Miller's image of an iceberg, is where masking takes place. "Masking hides the things below the water line," she says. "It hides specific triggers, so people aren't even aware of what's triggering their symptoms. The way patients describe this is, if they're living in a clean environment, as in Wimberley, and eating a safe diet, if a diesel truck drives by, they might notice specific symptoms associated with that truck. Headache, fatigue, nausea, depending on the individual. However, if they go to New York City, and they're staying in a hotel, and they're around fragrances, and there's a lot of auto exhaust, and suddenly a diesel truck drives by, they won't discern any relationship. Because there's so much background noise. In New York they're masked. In Wimberley they're de-masked."

And then jutting up above the water, either masked or demasked as the case may be (for the vast majority of MCS sufferers, it's almost certainly masked), is the rest of the iceberg, the symptoms from which the doctor makes a diagnosis.

Miller calls this theory Toxin-Induced Loss of Tolerance, or TILT. The acronym is conscious on Miller's part. She compares the onset of MCS to the workings of a pinball machine. "With a pinball machine, a player has just so much latitude — he can jiggle the machine, nudge it, bump it, rock it, but when he exceeds the limit for that machine, the "TILT" message appears, the lights go out, and the ball cascades to the bottom. The machine's tolerance has been exceeded and no amount of effort will make the bumpers or flippers operate as they did before. The game is over."

MCS sufferers hope the game isn't over. Fortunately, there are signs that for most it isn't. ("We help in excess of ninety percent of the patients we see," says Gerald Ross.) Why, then, this reluctance on the part of so many physicians even to consider the possibility that MCS may be other than a psychological problem? Because, Miller suggests, to do so would be to reject their training and best interests. "In recent times, many chronic diseases, addiction, and violence have been explained in whole or in part in terms of the psyche and stress," she declares. "An enormous amount of research has been devoted to these explanations. There are about thirty-seven thousand psychiatrists and two hundred forty thousand psychologists in the United States. Any theory of disease so bold as to suggest that depression, anxiety, panic attacks, or fatigue might be caused by chemical exposures should expect less than enthusiastic reception."

And there is the overwhelming influence of the pharmaceutical companies, the fragrance companies, the chemical companies, the very industrial basis of the developed world. The DuPont slogan — "Better Living Through Chemistry" — might just as well characterize this country's economy. A disease based on the contention that chemicals are bad for us threatens to unravel the fabric of our civilization — and the enormous profits gleaned from it. The commotion surrounding the tobacco industry's deceitful and intransigent response to widespread evidence of the health risks of smoking would be next to nothing compared to the uproar that would result from proof of chemical involvement in twentieth-century allergy.

* * *

But finally the brouhaha over MCS may boil down to a characteristic human tendency: we almost invariably try to resist change. We try to explain new problems by old models. Miller likes to quote MIT professor of philosophy Thomas Kuhn and his theories concerning the nature of scientific revolutions.

"Anomalies often pave the way for discovery," she explains. "The anomalous observation that individuals who survived a particular infection rarely contracted that infection again led to the immunologic concept of disease. The anomaly of MCS could likewise expand our thinking about disease causation. Thomas Kuhn observed that theories are 'generally preceded by a period of pronounced professional insecurity. As one might expect, that insecurity is generated by the persistent failure of the puzzles of normal science to come out as they should. Failure of existing rules is the prelude to a search for new ones.'

"Perhaps, we are in what Kuhn characterizes as a preparadigm period, a time 'regularly marked by frequent and deep debates over legitimate methods, problems, and standards of solution.'"

What, then, can people who suffer from multiple chemical sensitivity, and physicians who treat them do about resolving these debates? Until a definitive scientific marker for the illness comes along, something as demonstrable and widely accepted as a TB bacterium for TB, say, or until a treatment unambiguously and repeatedly relieves MCS's miseries, there may be nothing more to do than what people are now doing: trucking along as best they can and trying to spread the word in conferences such as the one in Princeton. But as I sit in the audience and listen to speaker after speaker contradict one another — indeed, not even appear to listen to one another — it seems hard to imagine that the lot of MCS sufferers may soon change.

Suddenly, in the middle of her talk, Miller flashes a slide on the screen. It's a quote from the German physicist Max Planck. She's not yet finished needling her colleagues.

"Scientific innovation rarely makes its way by gradually winning over and converting opponents. What does happen is that its opponents gradually die out."

If it is indeed a war of attrition, those who suffer from MCS may well hope that their opponents die out before they themselves do.

Chapter **6**

Fighting Back

WHEN KATIE CRECELIUS first began struggling to make a go of Ecology House, she knew she was in for a tough battle. "It's a complicated situation, largely because of two things," she says. "One, everybody is different. No two people react in quite the same way. Two, Ecology House is being used as an attention-getting mechanism, where chemically sensitive people feel that in order to get their rights recognized, they have to keep the MCS issue in the public eye."

Keeping MCS in the public eye — it's a vital strategy. If people who suffer from MCS are not to be ignored or labeled head cases or worse; if they are to make gains in the legislative arena; if they are to attract funding for mainstream medical research; in short, if they are to have any hope of improving their miserable fate, they must alert the world to the legitimacy of their cause.

That's where people like Mary Lamielle come in. Lamielle is an MCS activist, the founder and director of the National Center for Environmental Health Strategies (NCEHS). The title sounds grand; the reality is less imposing.

Drive down Lamielle's street in Vorhees Township, New Jersey, just outside Philadelphia, and you see a sedate, suburban neighborhood, "a very conservative neighborhood," says Lamielle. But Lamielle herself is anything but conservative, and her home is anything but sedate. Her home office — or anywhere in the house where there's a phone — is the headquarters of the NCEHS. And right now the phone is ringing. It seems as though it's always ringing. "Our center receives up to one thousand requests for information each month," Lamielle says. ("Our center" has a full-time staff of one — Lamielle herself.) Calls come from across the United States, Canada, New Zealand, Australia, Germany, and other countries. From the EPA, from Capitol Hill, from university researchers, from physicians, from chemically sensitive people complaining, questioning, cajoling, imploring. "I would estimate we've heard from fifteen thousand people with chemical sensitivity," she says. And from reporters, who know that Lamielle is a solid source of information and common sense.

Short and plump, with a round face and shaded eyeglasses framed in brown curls, Lamielle doesn't look the part of an activist. But she's forceful and fearless. She founded the NCEHS in 1986 as an outgrowth of her own frustrations. "Back in 'seventy-nine I was heading toward a doctorate in English," she says. "For a short time I also worked for the federal government. Then I went on a major downward health spiral." She's convinced that the primary reason involved a triple-whammy of exposures — to emissions from a malfunctioning sewage-treatment plant nearby; to odors of paint, wallpaper, new furniture, and carpeting from a remodeling project in her home; and to the pesticide Dursban, which Lamielle sprayed into her bedroom wall to get rid of a honeybee infestation. Lamielle soon found herself in a wheelchair, relying on oxygen to breathe. "I had flu-like symptoms constantly throughout the 'eighties, in addition to other symptoms that would come and go — chronic muscle and joint inflammation, for example. It took me till 'eighty-six to be able to function."

That's when she founded the NCEHS. She keeps it going, barely, through the kindness of strangers — that is, contributions. "So far I've worked out of my house, but we're desperately in need of an office," she says. "And we're desperate for money. We have a budget of thirty thousand dollars, but we never have more than a couple thousand dollars on hand. I'm very frustrated. A lot of our chemically sensitive people are very sick and may not have money, but it would be nice if somebody sent us a few bucks. We take advantage of community programs that have given us federally funded employees, but I haven't found a lot of helping hands. It's been a real struggle."

At first Lamielle concentrated on her organization's newsletter, *The Delicate Balance,* a dense collection of MCS news and tidbits that now makes its way to over four thousand subscribers. But more recently, as her health improved, she's been able to expand her reach. "It's only been in the last two and a half years that I've been physically out there testifying and lecturing," she says.

She does a lot of that. She has testified before Congress concerning the Indoor Air Quality Act. She has served as a member of the EPA's Lawn Care Pesticides Advisory Committee. She was instrumental in initiating one of the first comprehensive studies of MCS, a 1989 effort financed by the New Jersey Department of Health (it received an award from the World Health Organization). Written by Claudia Miller and MIT chemist and lawyer Nicholas Ashford, the study concluded that chemical sensitivity is "widespread in nature and is not limited to what some observers would describe as malingering workers, hysterical housewives, and workers experiencing psychogenic illness." While no definitive conclusions are yet possible, the study went on, "chemical sensitivity does exist as a serious health and environmental problem, and public and private sector action is warranted at both the state and federal levels." This was one of the first mainstream efforts to conclude that

MCS exists. In 1991 Ashford and Miller expanded it into the book *Chemical Exposures: Low Levels and High Stakes*, which John Selner blasted so bitterly.

In 1989, prompted in part by Lamielle's testimony, the Environmental Protection Agency's report to Congress on Indoor Air Quality mandated MCS research. Four years ago Congress designated $250,000 for the research, to be coordinated through the NCEHS. Although Lamielle's recommendations weren't faithfully followed, she's reasonably satisfied with the outcome. "Something is better than nothing," she says. "Some of the money was used to convene an expert panel to prioritize research issues. Money also went to fund a neuroscience workshop, and a piece of it went to California for recent work in diagnosing chemical sensitivity and tracking the exposure histories of people." But the NCEHS's primary recommendation, to fund an environmental unit, was ignored. "The money wasn't wasted in terms of beating the drum and getting this issue out there in the forefront, but I'm very frustrated. We're so far removed from having a unit. Without it, there's no foundation for valid research."

Lamielle serves on the expert panel convened by the Agency for Toxic Substances and Disease Registry to prioritize research issues. And in 1994 she was appointed to the President's Committee on Employment of People with Disabilities. She chairs a task force on MCS within the committee. One of her finest victories, however, has so far proven to be ironic. The 1990 Department of Housing and Urban Development (HUD) recognition of MCS as a disability is Lamielle's baby. "That's an area where we've worked hard to make things happen," she says. It was that act that made possible the noble experiment of Ecology House — and its disappointment and heartache.

Cynthia Wilson lives in the town of White Sulphur Springs, Montana. While she doesn't lobby Congress from that distant outpost, her Chemical Injury Information Network (CIIN) does offer free expert witness and doctor referrals, attorney referrals, referrals to less-toxic pesticide and weed-control experts and electromagnetic field experts, peer counseling, and materials for educational events. For a fee, CIIN will provide on-line literature searches and access to the organization's library. It also will provide a wide variety of articles having to do with MCS and other chemical-sensitivity issues. The latest order form I received lists 128 of them.

And CIIN offers a monthly newsletter. Called *Our Toxic Times,* it goes out to some five thousand members in the United States and twenty-nine other countries. It's a crisp little publication crammed with MCS information. Reprints of scientific papers, for example — "Neuropsychiatric Aspects of Sensitivity to Low-level Chemicals," by Iris Bell, is a recent one. A review of Claudia Miller's "Chemical Sensitivity Attributed to Pesticide Exposure Versus Remodeling" is another.

And another section, called "Did You Know?," offers short news blips. These are from January and February 1996:

- In 1989–90, 509,583 lbs. of malathion was used in Southern California to eradicate the medfly. It didn't work.
- Pesticide drift accounts for nearly 20% of all reported pesticide-related illnesses and injuries.
- In the first six months of 1995, the oil and coal industry made congressional re-election campaign contributions to the amount of $1.2 million.
- Prescription medicine dosage instructions are followed incorrectly by 30 to 50% of patients.
- 22 different insecticides, including DDT and Chlordane, were found in 200 samples of tree bark taken from 90 sites worldwide.
- Women are 3 times more likely to have children who get leukemia if they are exposed to pesticides during pregnancy.

- Pesticides are believed to cause at least 20,000 cases of cancer each year.

Perhaps the most interesting parts of the newsletter, however, are the ads. They go a long way toward characterizing the unnatural everyday reality of MCS, a reality in which the simplest and most common implements of life are fraught with danger.

100% Cotton Shower Curtain!
(Just say nope* to vinyl)

Your plastic liner off-gasses chemicals that can make you sick. **Replace it with our 100% COTTON untreated liner today!** Tightly woven cotton duck gets wet, but water stays in the tub. No liner necessary. Machine washable! Rustproof brass grommets. Natural color, treated only with cornstarch sizing (which comes out in first washing). $35 + $3.75 shipping. Send check to . . .

*nope (nonpolluting enterprises)

Hygenaire~TM~

The air we breathe indoors should be the cleanest air available. Clean air doesn't just happen, it takes *air care.* HYGENAIRE's all natural botanical ingredients will neutralize odors before they become a problem.

Odors originate from many biological sources, as in the picture below. Put out a protective barrier against odors and breathe easier. HYGENAIRE is the first of a new generation of air fresheners that improve indoor air quality.

Imagine having clean, odor-free air, using no masking fragrances or cover-up scents, ozone, or filtration. Designed and extensively tested by people with Environmental Illness and Multiple Chemical Sensitivity, HYGENAIRE is an effective and safe alternative to other air treatments.

CHEMICAL-FREE
LAUNDRY ALTERNATIVE

REUSABLE LAUNDRY DISCS
Wash Your Clothes Clean Without Detergent!
A Revolutionary New Way to Clean Your Clothes!

The Discs . . .

- **Work without soaps, detergents, or chemicals.**
- Need no fabric softener or static-cling sheets.
- Do not pollute waste water.
- Kill various types of bacteria.
- Are easy to use — no spills of powders or liquids.
- Clean a typical family's laundry for approximately
  2 years — about 700 loads of laundry.
- Have a 30-day unconditional money-back guarantee.

Set of 3 Reusable Laundry Discs
Just $49.95

Products for the Chemically Sensitive
& Environmentally Aware

Are You Sensitive to Chemicals?

Consider AFM Safecoat and SafeChoice — the leader in building and maintenance products for the chemically sensitive for 15 years.

Significant features and benefits when using AFM's Safecoat and SafeChoice Products:

- Reduce Toxic Emissions
- Low or No Odor
- Low or Zero VOC

- A full line of products recommended by Environmental Physicians.
- 12-year history of successful use by the "chemically sensitive"

Over 35 products for safer indoor environments:
1) Paints, coatings & stains
2) Cleaning & maintenance
3) Carpet Maintenance
4) Adhesive . . . and More!

Environmentally Safe House
for Sale in Wisconsin

3-bedroom, 2-bath ranch, hardwood and ceramic floors,
all electric, 3/4 acre lot, organic garden.
Located on a quiet street.

E.I. Safe Townhouse

Washington, D.C., area (Md.)
Hardwood Floors • Hypoallergenic Paint • No Spraying on Either Side
Would consider renting

PESTICIDE
FREE

FOR RENT

EXTREMELY SAFE Porcelain Trailer on 10 acres in Northern Arizona.
Safe Washer & Dryer Available. $450 per month plus electricity

PESTICIDE
FREE

Homeless MCS Woman has found a donor of a safe
trailer. We need help to transport it over 1,500 miles.
Can you help us with a donation? Checks may be made
payable to . . .

Heavenly Heat
Sauna rooms

Specializing in safe home saunas for the chemically sensitive.
From economical personal units to family-sized rooms.
All models can be disassembled and moved.
Serving the needs of the environmentally sensitive community.
"Sweat It Out!"

Chadwick's
Chemically Sensitive
Salon

Offering healthful
hair care in the safest
environment possible

Accommodation/Benefits Representation

Retired Civil Rights attorney will represent claimants at
Social Security, HUD, EEOC hearings.
Experienced in ADA, IDEA, Rehabilitation Act, etc.

HELP COPING WITH
INDOOR AIR POLLUTION

We can help you cope with indoor air pollution due
to perfumes, air fresheners, copy machines, marking
pens, carbonless paper, carpets, insulation, etc. —
Telephone consultations at $25 per quarter hour.

Homeopathic and Herbal Medicines

Medicine for the 21st Century. Be a part of it.
Help others. Become a Nature's Sunshine distributor of
Homeopathic and Herbal medicines. Call or write . . .

How long has it been since you've been able to eat Gummy Bears?

I've found a Gummy Bear which is equal
to 1 serving of fruits and
vegetables in a vegetable gelatin base.
CONTAINS NO CORN SYRUP,
ARTIFICIAL COLORING,
OR FLAVORING

For more details, call . . .

Albert Donnay doesn't have to use any of these products. The difference between him and Wilson, Lamielle, and just about every other MCS activist is this: Donnay does not suffer from multiple chemical sensitivity.

"Thank God!" he exclaims. "That's one of the problems in this field — the patients are so sick they can't get anything done. It's been astounding how many of them cannot believe that there's a healthy person working on this."

In 1993, Donnay, a master's degree recipient from the Johns Hopkins School of Hygiene and Public Health and an experienced environmental health researcher, was tapped by Baltimore environmental physician Grace Ziem as a research associate. Soon they founded MCS Referral & Resources, initially to promote and distribute educational materials for Ziem's own patients, but increasingly to reach the rest of the world. Sufferer or no, the lightning-quick, fast-talking Donnay has become a dedicated MCS activist.

The fact that he's healthy isn't the only difference between him and the others. Whereas MCS-sufferer activists tend to weigh their words carefully lest they publicly offend others in this contentious field, Donnay is exuberantly outspoken. And never more so than on the subject of what he considers the Machiavellis in the MCS world: industry-supported physician-apologists. The snakes in the grass whose credentials provide respectability but whose agenda is determined by their financial supporters. The nature of their agenda? To discredit MCS.

There is no doubt that in the background of the MCS story lurks the unsettling specter of money. Money, and the people who make it and defend it. For what is the source of multiple chemical sensitivity? Pesticides, common household cleaners, building materials, perfumes, deodorants, vehicle exhaust — the products of industry. "If you go to any major meeting on chemical sensitivity, there are representatives from the perfume, carpet, and chemical industries," says Claudia Miller. "They're extremely concerned about the outcome of this debate."

That's where Ronald Gots comes in. Gots (who explained the similarities between MCS and autointoxication; see chapter 4) is an active player in the drama. As one of the most vocal of those who insist on the psychogenic origin of MCS, Gots provides the chemical industry just what it needs: public assurance that whatever else might be going on in MCS, chemicals have nothing to do with it.

"If you define the problem as people who develop symptoms to what they *believe* are chemical exposures, then, absolutely, there are those people," Gots says. "But if you define it as an organically based process whereby chemicals somehow physically alter the body and cause an ailment, I don't think there's any evidence for that. I think it's a group of psychologically derived phenomena.

"Multiple chemical sensitivities is a dangerous diagnosis," he goes on. "Unlike many 'alternative medical practices,' the diagnosis of MCS begins a downward spiral of fruitless treatments, culminating in withdrawal from society and condemning the sufferer to a life of misery and disability. This is a phenomenon in which the diagnosis is far more disabling than the symptoms.

"The MCS theory . . . has generally been rejected as a 'junk science,'" Gots contends.

Donnay considers all that pure bunk. "It's such a shame that the myth is still out there that there's nothing to this disease," he declares. "The myth dates to the late eighties and early nineties, when a few medical societies issued negative opinions that were strongly influenced by their anti-MCS expert witness members, who pushed for these statements so they could use them in court. People like Gots.

"But one of the first things I did when I got this job was a literature search. Our database goes back to 1954 — over three hundred references, more than half of them written since the last medical society opinion was issued in 1992, categorized as to whether they support a psychological basis, organic basis, or both. The trend is two to one physiological over psychological. There are only ten studies of actual patients that claim to have found a psychological basis, and a Hopkins researcher looked at them and found that all of them had fundamental methodological errors. So there's really no strength at all to the scientific evidence suggesting it's psychological. And in addition to all the papers on the other side, over a hundred and fifty suggesting it's physiological, there's the involvement of half a dozen federal agencies sponsoring over half a dozen scientific conferences on MCS in the last five years. Nineteen federal agencies that have recognized MCS. Six Canadian authorities that have recognized MCS. Nineteen U.S. state authorities. Eleven U.S. local authorities. Nineteen independent organizations and institutions. All that tells me that despite what Gots says, this is not a fringe, unrecognized disorder. All this wouldn't be happening if this were a non-disease and a non-issue."

Donnay is trying to expose Gots's organization, the Environmental Sensitivities Research Institute, ESRI, as little more than an industry mouthpiece rather than the research- and education-oriented nonprofit association it claims to be. "We know that they've been going with their hand out to various industry trade associations," he says. "Carpet industry, pesticide industry, drug industry, perfume industry, insurance industry. So many industries are affected by MCS, so many that he can sell his science spin services to."

Those services do not come cheap. Gots's ESRI offers two member categories: Enterprise Membership at $10,000 annually, and Service Membership at $5,000. Gots claims that anyone is welcome to join, but fees like that restrict membership to people or organizations with deep pockets and vested interests. (Compare to Cynthia Wilson's yearly rates of $10 to $15 for people with fixed incomes, $25 to $30 for individuals, and $50 to $75 for professionals for her Chemical Injury Information Network, which provides several of the same services as Gots's organizations — but for people on the other side of the battlefield. In this war, money alone guarantees an unequal fight.)

Combine the ESRI with another of Gots's organizations, the National Medical Advisory Service, which provides expert witnesses to attorneys defending corporations in product liability lawsuits — a frequent occupation of Gots himself — and you've got a potent double-whammy of anti-MCS testimony. "And they're both under the same roof," says Donnay. "There's not a very fine distinction there. Unfortunately he's rarely called on it."

One of the most insidious of Gots's actions in Donnay's view was his presentation of the U.S. position on MCS in a February 1996 meeting sponsored by the International Program on Chemical Safety (IPCS), the result of which was a recommendation that the term "multiple chemical sensitivity" be scrapped in favor of "idiopathic environmental intolerances" (IEI). "Idiopathic" means "a disease of unknown origin or cause." IEI, then, suggests that the disorder is *associated with* everyday environmental factors tolerated by the majority of people but has no known cause. In other words, there is no identifiable culprit — and that lets chemical industries off the hook. The term "IEI" suggests that people who claim suffering may well be creating their own misery.

Well, that made Donnay furious. All the more so because he discovered that of seventeen invited "experts" who participated in the conference, only seven had ever published anything related to MCS. Others shared his outrage. Soon after the IPCS recommendations came out, a group of more than sixty occupational and environmental health scientists from around the world signed a letter of protest that was sent to IPCS and its three United Nations sponsors. Among other things, the letter stated that "IPCS has demonstrated extreme bias in favor of the chemical and asbestos industries in its evaluations of environmental health hazards to the public. Immediate, comprehensive steps need to be taken to restore the credibility of IPCS, and, by implication, the United Nations sponsors of IPCS (World Health Organization, International Labor Office, United Nations Environment Program)."

The scientists urged the IPCS to "immediately halt work toward the issuance of reports on Multiple Chemical Sensitivities. Reconstitute the MCS panel exclusively with scientists who have published research (not merely opinion) on chemical sensitivity and related scientific issues and with doctors who have actual experience in managing patients with Multiple Chemical Sensitivities . . . and to the fullest extent possible identify and exclude scientists with financial conflicts of interest."

And they demanded that the IPCS "report publicly on the complete extent of conflicts of interest of all members of IPCS expert scientific panels."

"That was an amazing coup," Donnay says. "We rarely see that kind of activism among professional scientists. Yet they all felt strongly enough about what IPCS had done to sign that letter."

In August Donnay circulated to the media and government officials a document entitled "Undisclosed Bias and Misrepresentations of Dr. Ronald Gots." In it he revealed that Gots has been testifying as a paid witness against MCS since at least 1985, representing Dow Chemical among other clients; that ESRI, his *research* institute, does not actually do any research; that its board of directors includes representatives of Procter & Gamble; the Cosmetic, Toiletry and Fragrance Association; Monsanto; and Dow-Elanco, "the manufacturer of chlorpyrifos (aka Dursban), which is associated with more reports of chemical sensitivity than any other pesticide"; and that while Gots claims he is a toxicologist, his Ph.D. is actually in pharmacology, his training in surgery, and he has not treated a patient in more than 20 years. Moreover, while he readily speaks out against MCS, he has published only three opinion articles, none based on any original research.

A response wasn't long in coming. In September Donnay received a letter from Gots's attorney, demanding that he terminate his campaign to defame Gots. Gots does sound scientific research; Donnay's statements are nothing but personal attacks.

Donnay's response was even swifter. Nine days later he wrote back. Everything I've said about Gots is true, he stated. Far from circulating false statements, I want to correct *Gots's* false and misleading statements. And until you prove otherwise, I'm going to keep on doing it!

And so the matter remains. Gots continues to offer his opinions on MCS, Donnay continues to attack them. "I'm going to see what we can push the Maryland state attorney general's office to reveal about ESRI." He laughs in disgust and exasperation. "It's an amazing group."

If vested interests are implicit in the activities of MCS naysayers like Ronald Gots, they seem all too obvious in the sad case of *Rogers vs. Benjamin Moore, et al.* The plaintiff: Texas housewife Connie Rogers. The defendants: Benjamin Moore & Company and some two dozen other contractors and building material manufacturers. The setting: the hill country haven for MCS sufferers, Wimberley, Texas.

The first inkling that something was very wrong came in February of 1988, when the Wimberley Independent School District held an open house for its brand-new Scudder Elementary School. The school seemed to be under a cloud — or, as Connie Rogers might say, a curse. At the open house one parent started vomiting, another suffered a nosebleed. A child became nauseated, and another broke out with red splotches all over her body. Over the next few weeks of school more children began dropping. One developed profuse nosebleeds, another a rash, another lost five pounds in two days, another developed hives so severe she couldn't stand to wear clothes. When Rogers's five-year-old son, Dusty, came home from his first day at kindergarten, "his ears were so red, they looked like they were bleeding. His whole nose was burnt tissue. We had to put topical painkillers in his nose and ears," she says. And his sister, Dallas, developed nosebleeds and a croup-like cough.

Over time, between thirty-six and sixty-eight sick kids had to be pulled out of a school that had only three hundred children enrolled in the first place. And soon it was disclosed that the materials used to build the school contained formaldehyde and hydrocarbons, among other toxic substances. The school gave every indication of being a particularly potent "sick building."

Sue Pitman saw it coming. "In 1987 I came back from my Christmas holiday to see in the newspaper that there had been a meeting of the school board about building a new elementary school out of Styrofoam," she says. "It had to be a joke. So I called the local dentist, who was on the school board, and who had treated chemically sensitive people. He knew what all this was about. He said, 'You better find out all you can about this building material.'"

The building material did indeed turn out to be Styrofoam, enormous wedges of it, sandwiched between huge pieces of particle board–like panels. The result was an instant, prefab building. The brand name was Futurebuilt.

"So I checked around," Pitman says. "I called Dr. Rea's office and found out that several of their patients had had their chemical sensitivities triggered in such buildings. I got the school board to have an environmental consultant review the plans and specs. She said that if they built it, it was going to be one of the most toxic buildings anywhere. The whole thing got to be very controversial in town, because the architect who was proposing to build with this material was connected to Futurebuilt."

The warring parties met privately in the town library. "It was a nasty meeting," remembers Pitman. "The architect just ran all over the consultant, said that her recommendations were a bunch of hogwash, they couldn't change things, it would wreck the building."

Then came a large public meeting. "My final argument had been to at least build an adequate ventilation system," Pitman says. "And some other parents wanted no carpets. I remember the school board president saying, in front of all these people, 'Sue, we can argue about this forever . . .' So they built the school, pretty much as designed."

Then came the fateful open house. Sue Pitman didn't attend — "I had no desire to go there. I was getting well. I don't take chances like that."

And neither did Connie Rogers. "I didn't even know about the open house," she says. "And I didn't really pay attention to what happened. I thought it was all pretty silly. I just thought, 'Well, they'll open the windows, open the doors, and it'll air out.'"

In fact, Rogers hadn't paid attention to the school controversy from the beginning. Nor had she paid attention to the problem of multiple chemical sensitivity. She didn't suffer the malady, didn't know anyone who did, didn't travel in those circles. She wouldn't go near a clinical ecologist if you paid her. She was no desperate chemical refugee to the area. She was a native, a Texan born and bred.

"I'm an *old* American," she says. "My family is original Texas land grants, the people before the *Mayflower*." Rogers *sounds* like an original Texan, with a lively twang and a bent for colorful language. "I am definitely a bubba-ette. A bubba-ette is someone who can handle bubbas. I'm the one who can wrangle them." What she couldn't wrangle was what happened to her kids.

Soon after the open house, the school opened for business. But it was hardly ready. "They occupied it before it was finished," Rogers says. "There was no sewage system, just an open septic tank that had a ten-foot drop with no fence around it. There was no grass. There was no kitchen. Most of the plumbing didn't work. They were still laying down carpet, still painting, still putting cabinets up. They were still laying tile, still putting adhesive down. They were using the gymnasium as a storage room, and the kids would pile on top of these panels and carpet pieces which were heavily treated. They were gluing carpet panels on the walls for soundboards while the kids were already in the classrooms. They were still hooking up a telephone the first day they let them in. And the ventilation system was so poor. It's incredible how bad it was. The kids weren't getting any fresh air. There was just a two-inch pipe to feed each classroom. That's all the air they got. That and a small window.

"I still don't know why they put the children in an incomplete school. There wasn't but three months left of the semester anyway. It seemed quite stupid to move these children into a school that wasn't finished."

It was then that Rogers's son, Dusty, came home sick. "Within hours of being in the school, his ears were infected, his throat, his nose," she recalls. "We were putting painkillers in his ears and nose to numb 'em because they were burning. But we just thought, 'Well, it's a virus that's going around. Everybody has this bug.'"

But the bug, if that's what it was, didn't go away. "I called around and got the names of people who thought that their kids were sick," says Sue Pitman. "I did a little survey and found that eighteen percent of kids in the school felt like they were being affected by the fumes, some more severely than others."

"The school people, they'd say, 'Oh, well, kids get nosebleeds,'" Rogers recalls. "But twenty kids in one day don't usually get nosebleeds. Twenty kids don't usually start vomiting. The custodians were constantly cleaning up. They were getting upset."

As for Dusty, "He just kept getting sicker and sicker. He would get very lethargic and nauseated. He couldn't eat." And Dallas, her daughter, developed hearing and respiratory problems.

The situation came to a head a couple of months later, when Rogers's sister, who was working at the school as a custodian, went into Dusty's classroom. "She unlocked the door and found him lying on the carpet, swollen, gasping," Rogers says. As one of Dusty's symptoms during this siege was hyperactivity, the teacher was punishing him by making him stay inside while all the other kids went out to play. Without knowing any better, she was denying him the very thing that would have helped him most — fresh air, getting away from the building.

"My sister picked him up and called me immediately," says Rogers. "That was the last time he was ever at the school.

"I had tried to stay away from the controversy. But I realized that I was gonna have to deal with what was wrong with my son. I was trying to figure out what it was, and someone said, 'I know a lady ...'"

And so, native Texan "bubba-ette" Connie Rogers teamed up with chemically sensitive émigré Sue Pitman. "From then on, what she said made sense," says Rogers. "My son had developed into a bed wetter. And when I say 'bed wetter,' I don't mean that he wet the bed, we'd get up and change him, and everything was fine. I mean he would wet the bed two and three times during the night, plus get up and go to the bathroom. Well, I went kind of crazy. I just didn't know what was what. Sue came over and found that the bed had a polystyrene mattress, with foam in his pillows. I even had a plastic cover under his sheet so he wouldn't ruin the bed. His room was decorated up in vinyl sharks and things. I was doing everything wrong. We got rid of all of it, and we brought in a cotton mattress that I had slept on as a child and replaced the bed with a metal bedframe. I took all the carpet out of the house, all the curtains out of the house, all his toys out. The house was basically stripped down. It's ceramic-tiled now, with Portland cement. We took great pains trying to set up a perfect world for him, or near as close to a glass bubble as we could get. And the bed-wetting stopped."

What made the whole business even worse was that the school didn't seem to care. "For a while the school begrudgingly provided alternative classrooms," says Pitman. "The kids whose parents were concerned were put in a room in the old elementary school, ostracized from the other kids, where they were essentially baby-sat rather than instructed. That lasted for a couple weeks."

The doctor in town didn't understand what was going on. The state health department didn't know what to do. And woe be to anyone who criticized the status quo. Says Pitman: "If you said anything about your kids being sick in the school, that was an attack on the school district, an attack on the social structure of the community. It got very personal."

Finally, Connie Rogers and her compatriots took out their frustration and anger in the only way that seemed left to them: they filed a lawsuit charging product liability, fraud, and negligence against nearly two dozen contractors and building manufacturers. *Rogers vs. Benjamin Moore, et al.* involved forty-three children and forty-two adults asking almost $4 billion from such giants as Benjamin Moore & Co., Ashland Chemical, Inc., and BASF Corp.

"I filed the lawsuit to recoup the loss for the taxpayers so that we could get the school fixed," Rogers says. "If we won, the children would keep their money, and the adults would put their money over to fixing the school. So it wouldn't cost the taxpayers anything."

"Did you really ask for *four billion?*" I ask.

"I wasn't after *that* much. The lawyers set that."

But if Rogers and the others involved thought that filing the lawsuit might ease their pain, all it did was make things worse. They became *personae non gratae* in their own town.

"She filed suit because there was no other recourse," says Pitman. "It was a problem, it was wrong, and it needed to be addressed. But people kept thinking, or were led to believe, that she was suing the school, which was like suing the community. Which she never did. She sued the people who provided the toxic building materials."

No matter. Rogers became a target for the town's indignation and lack of understanding. "I'm a vocal person," she says.

"I definitely speak my mind, and I won't step away from a fight. Unfortunately, people like to threaten you in the grocery store. They would do small things like ram you with their basket. They would throw meat at you. Scratch your car. Follow you in the dark with no lights on to scare you. They would make obscene phone calls. They threatened to poison your well. They threatened to burn your house down. They actually cut one of the mothers' brake lines."

Sue Pitman corroborates these incidents. "Connie'd walk into a movie theater, and people would get up and leave. Once she went to a school game at the Wimberley stadium, and people were making loud, obnoxious, abusive comments. And it's true about the brakes of one of the mothers. The repair person said it looked like the brake lines had been cut almost all the way through. She had been a Realtor in the community, and had a lot of good friends. When people began turning against her, it became real difficult."

Finally, Connie Rogers had a nervous breakdown punctuated by recurrent nightmares about the experience. In August of 1995, the Rogers family moved away from Wimberley. And seven years after it had been filed, *Rogers vs. Benjamin Moore, et al.* was settled out of court. "They settled, but they settled as a nuisance," Rogers says. "There was no precedent set, there was nothing. It was just quietly pushed off. The children got a nominal amount — you couldn't buy a car with it. It was nothing compared to what my son had gone through."

Rogers blames her attorneys. And she blames what more than one person involved regards as a conspiracy among the Wimberley establishment to cover up an intricate web of double-dealing and profiteering among school board members, lawyers, bankers, politicians, contractors, and building material suppliers — a number of whom wore more than one hat in the enterprise.

"The bank president, the local lawyers, the PTA — these people were on the school board," Rogers says. "The money people were on the school board. They had a vested interest in the school. They didn't want to hear anything that threatened their investment in the school. They built this school for 1.8 million dollars. If they would have built the same school out of cinderblock, it woulda only cost eight hundred thousand. You tell me what's wrong with this picture."

"Did these same people have an interest in the construction company?" I ask. I had heard rumors that one of the assets alluded to in the divorce papers of a school board member was stock in Futurebuilt and that the local bank came close to being indicted for shady business dealings surrounding the construction of the school.

"Who knows?" Rogers replies. "The bank financed building the school. And the bank president . . . well, he blew his brains out."

Today Dusty Rogers still suffers repercussions from those times. But he's doing better. And so is his mother. She still has nightmares about the experience, but now she's able to talk about it. "We still live in Texas, but I don't want anybody to know where. We live in the hill country, *way* in the hill country. It's a little isolated town. Bubbaville. We live right by the river. It's nice. You can walk down and watch the ducks."

Connie Rogers is not the only one suing. As far back as 1979 people claiming to suffer from MCS have been going to court to demand compensation, with varying results. But no matter their outcome, court battles such as these offer yet another stage for the antipathy between traditional and alternative physicians to play itself out. "A lot of mainstream physicians, allergists included, have served as expert witnesses for the defense in cases where MCS patients have alleged they are sick," says Claudia Miller. "MCS patients will present data from ecologists, and the traditionally trained allergists will say, 'That stuff doesn't make sense. It's not accepted medical practice.'

The deck is stacked against the patients. And when you have on the defense side the classical allergists and occupational health doctors, and on the plaintiff side the clinical ecologists, the debate becomes even more emotional and vitriolic."

Such ill will doesn't deter Al Levin one whit. Levin revels in taking on the world. In his view, however, the proper target is not a warring medical community but rather the powers behind it.

"If you have a controversy, there's got to be something fueling the fire," he says. "So you look behind the traditional allergists and whom do you see? Drug companies, chemical companies, food companies. And whom do you see behind them? The same people who gave us the Vietnam War.

"Hughes Industries runs the largest research programs of Harvard, Hopkins, UCSF. McDonnell-Douglas runs seventy-five percent of all hardware and software of all the hospitals in this country. Lockheed owns Dialogue Database, the biggest, best medical database in the country. FMC, which makes tanks and armored vehicles, has a contract with Hybrotech, a biotech company that makes monoclonal antibodies. Colt Industries has a division that does automated urinalysis. You can go on and on and on. These defense contractors went into medicine with exactly the same ethics that they had in Vietnam. *None!*

"So what happens is that when a group of doctors say that the products of these contractors can cause illness, these contractors hire other doctors to disqualify them. To take their license away. Same thing that happened in the military. Same people, same everything. The world continues to turn, and everything that goes around comes around. There's a battle here."

But it's an unequal battle. The big guns are all on one side. Levin's strategy for fighting the fight, therefore, is simple: use the same tactics the other side uses.

"In 1981 I went to the clinical ecologists' meeting in Banff, Alberta. They had about seven, eight thousand dollars to spend. They wanted to know what kind of research protocol they could put together to prove that clinical ecology is a valid medical discipline. I got up and said, 'Look, you got to understand — there's no proof that anything is a valid medical discipline. It depends on who's supporting it. If you have a dollar to spend on research and a dollar to spend on a politician, you buy the politician. Let's forget about the science. That's baloney.'"

As evidence, Levin points to a famous incident in the history of medicine, the Flexner Report of 1910. At the turn of the century American medicine was a hodgepodge of different approaches. Present-day "alternative" disciplines such as homeopathy, naturopathy, and osteopathy flourished side by side with allopathy, the method we've come to regard as orthodox medicine.

The Flexner Report went a long way to change all that. In 1908 an obscure educator named Abraham Flexner (his brother, Simon, was the well-known head of the Rockefeller Institute in Manhattan) was commissioned by the Carnegie Foundation, acting on an invitation from the Council of Medical Education of the American Medical Association, a five-man committee of university-educated physicians, to carry out a review of medical education in this country. There were some 150 medical schools at the time. Flexner visited them all. He concluded that medical education in America was a mess and should be standardized. It should be provided by a university-based, research-oriented medical school along the lines of the paragon of turn-of-the-century American medicine, Johns Hopkins in Baltimore. It should be properly equipped with laboratories and wards, like Hopkins, should admit only academically qualified students, like Hopkins, and, like Hopkins, should emphasize original research. Doctoring should be a scientific discipline that required extensive clinical training through at least a year of internship. A fledgling doc anywhere in the country would have available the same body of knowledge as a trainee at Hopkins itself.

Given the influence of the work of Pasteur, Lister, and Koch, which had been filtering out of Europe for three decades, that Flexner leaned in this direction is not surprising, And it is not surprising given the fact that the impetus for commissioning the report in the first place had come from the AMA's cadre of university medical people, who in 1906, without publishing the information, had themselves conducted a similar investigation that came to similar conclusions. "As it seemed politically imprudent for a medical organization to be so publicly critical of medical schools, the council invited the Carnegie Foundation for the Advancement of Teaching to conduct a similar study," reads an inquiry into the development of American medicine. One can imagine that the council was hardly upset by Flexner's recommendations.

The event is often considered the beginning of modern medicine. As soon as the report came out, it was strongly backed by all major national associations, including the AMA (reluctantly, however, as most of its members were non-university educated practicing docs, who had little to do with the organization's university physicians) and all university-based hospitals, in particular the influential Eastern institutions, Hopkins in the lead. Over the next five years, 60 percent of all American medical schools folded. Those that survived adopted the Hopkins model.

Levin considers the effects of this turnaround to be of mixed value — and not necessarily the result of open-minded investigation. "Flexner said that naturopaths and homeopaths were practicing unscientific medicine and so their schools should be shut down," Levin explains. "And allopaths had to have a uniform curriculum, so that somebody studying in Boston and somebody studying in St. Louis would know the same thing.

"All that sounds good on the surface. But at that point

preventive medicine, nutrition, and all those things that aren't good for business became unimportant classes in medical school. Big-dollar things like surgery, internal medicine, and pharmacology became very important." In other words, the new dispensation in medicine favored high-tech procedures and the dispensing of drugs. That meant big bucks for big business.

In Levin's eyes, then, the resulting bias as to what is good medicine and what is not has had obvious ramifications for MCS and environmental physicians. And for him the reality that medicine is controlled by big business rather than medical interests explains why the papers published in mainstream journals almost always refute the possible chemical basis of MCS.

"Almost all the advertising in the *New England Journal of Medicine* comes from drug companies," says Levin. "So you're not going to say anything bad about their products. You have to be awfully naive to think that the *New England Journal* is going to publish something that's adverse to their advertisers. I have a friend who was a senior editor for JAMA. She wrote an article on a calcium channel blocker that was better than one of the calcium channel blockers advertised in the journal. She was called in to write a retraction. She refused, and she was out of a job."

For Levin, all this is simply the way the world works, and the sooner environmental physicians face reality, the better off they, and their patients, will be. "These people who get righteously indignant and say, 'This is unfair, this is dishonest' . . . Give me a break! You need money, you need power. I tried to tell the clinical ecologists that at their meeting, and they just laughed at me. Booed me off the podium. But I defend them vigorously. Because they're absolutely right."

And when Levin says "defend them," he means *defend* them. A few years ago he went back to school — to law school — and in the spring of 1995 he received his law degree. In December he was admitted to the California Bar, and in the spring of 1996 to the Texas Bar. With the help of Bill Rea and other physicians testifying as expert witnesses, Levin has big plans.

"I'm going to reform American medicine," he declares. "I have a lot of contacts on all sides. I'm going to get 'em, and they're going to squeal. All the way up."

Chapter 7

Storm from the Desert

YOU WOULDN'T THINK that Gary Zuspann and Jerry Phillips had much in common. Jerry is forty-eight years old, six feet tall, and a thick 250 pounds in a black T-shirt and jeans. Short-cropped brown hair, short-cropped brown beard, on his left forearm a tattoo with a smirking devil encircled by the words, "Born To Raise Hell." You wouldn't want to run into Jerry in a dark alley. You wouldn't be surprised to see Jerry pull away in a big rig or on a Harley.

Gary, thirty-six years old, is six foot, three inches, and bone-thin. His longish, receding black hair frames a pale, gentle, al-most childlike face. He wears glasses, sports a stubble of black beard. He slumps in a wheelchair, an oxygen mask pressed to his nose and mouth. The Boy Scout next door. The sickly Sun-day school teacher. The innocent victim.

So much for differences. The similarities are more pro-found. Both Gary and Jerry are Gulf War vets. And both of them are ill. Both of them are here at the Environmental Health Center in Dallas for checkups. Both of them are casual-ties of what, for lack of a better term, has been dubbed Gulf War syndrome, or GWS.

* * *

The Persian Gulf War lasted little more than a month — from January 16 to February 27, 1991. Of the seven hundred thousand U.S. troops sent to the Gulf fewer than three hundred died; barely four hundred were wounded. By comparison, estimates are that one hundred thousand Iraqi soldiers were killed, three hundred thousand were wounded, one hundred fifty thousand deserted, and sixty thousand were taken prisoner. Most observers consider the war an overwhelming coalition victory, even more decisive, and much quicker, than anticipated.

What wasn't anticipated, however, were the reports of strange maladies afflicting returning troops. Fatigue, diarrhea, skin rashes, muscle and joint pain, headaches, loss of memory, difficulty breathing, gastrointestinal and respiratory problems, and worse. Some veterans reported the identical illnesses in their spouses and children, as though whatever it was that struck them was contagious. Some vets even reported birth defects in children conceived after their return. A study conducted by former senator Donald Riegle Jr. of Michigan found that 78 percent of veterans' wives were afflicted with the same problems as their husbands, as were 65 percent of children born to them after their return. Ellen Silbergeld, a molecular toxicologist at the University of Maryland, told a 1994 congressional hearing that men exposed to toxic chemicals can pass on genetic mutations to their children via their sperm.

To date, more than eighty thousand vets have registered with the Veterans Administration (VA) as suffering from Gulf War syndrome and some thirty thousand more with the Department of Defense (DOD). Many of them consider their symptoms a legacy of the precautions against biological and chemical attack they were encouraged to take before deploying to the Gulf. Many others feel they were made sick by the very conditions they were trying to protect against: toxic fumes, pesticides, local microbes, chemical warfare. And in this war, for the first time, tens of thousands of anti-tank uranium-tipped shells were used. A confidential 1991 report from the British Atomic Energy Authority to the Ministry of Defense warned that the forty tons of depleted uranium dust left on the battlefield could, in theory, cause half a million deaths.

But as far as the Pentagon is concerned, there is no such thing as Gulf War syndrome. An $80 million, two-year Department of Defense study released in April of 1996 found, in the words of Assistant Secretary of Defense for Health Affairs Stephen Joseph, "no indication of a unique illness, or a Persian Gulf syndrome or a single entity, that would account for illness in any large or significant fraction of these . . . people."

Rather, according to Joseph, Gulf War syndrome is a mix of various problems from various sources. There are "musculo-skeletal conditions" — acquiring "a bad hip from falling off the back of a Hummvee," for example. There are "ill-defined conditions" — "diseases that would have developed anyway, whether they had gone to the Gulf or whether they had stayed in San Diego." And there are "psychological conditions." These are the primary source of the vets' troubles. Says Joseph, "Our data show that the largest single category of diagnoses are psychological ones." Most likely it's all in their heads.

Moreover, these maladies were to be expected. They're par for the course, nothing to get alarmed about. "When you send a large number of healthy young people off into an extremely dangerous and stressful environment, surprise, surprise, some proportion of them come home with a variety of illnesses," says Joseph. "I think if you look at a population of healthy young people who go off to war in a very hostile environment, which it always is, you would see something like this."

Sound familiar? A variety of debilitating symptoms, perhaps associated with exposure to chemicals, branded most likely the result of psychogenic problems. Gulf War syndrome is the wild card in the multiple chemical sensitivity story. In an ironic way, this controversial outbreak may actually be a lucky break for those suffering MCS.

Of course, the Phillips and Zuspann families don't see things quite that way. Maybe because Jerry and Gary's collection of so-called musculoskeletal conditions, psychological conditions, and ill-defined conditions have torn apart their lives. Their stories are harrowing.

"I'm a Vietnam vet," Jerry says. "I was working as a mechanic for the Oklahoma National Guard. We took care of three hundred pieces of rolling stock in Ardmore, Oklahoma, a hundred miles north of Dallas. All my life I've either been a mechanic or truck driver. I've worked around solvents and paints and chemicals all my life. I never had no problem with them."

In December of 1990, Jerry was mobilized to active duty. Before going overseas to Saudi Arabia, he and the rest of his unit received a battery of inoculations. "They put us in a line, said, 'You have to get this, this, this,'" Jerry recalls. "But they didn't tell us what we were getting."

Soon he was admitted to the emergency room with a high fever and congestion. The diagnosis was pneumonia. "We were put in old World War Two barracks," Jerry recalls. "The showers and bathrooms were not in the building. They were in a separate building out on the parade field. It was cold enough that the water would freeze in the toilets. If you had to go to the bathroom, you would have to walk a hundred yards to the toilet and back. You'd have to walk to the shower and back. We thought I got sick because of the cold, but now we're not sure."

On New Year's Eve Jerry shipped out, his destination Jabal, a large port city south of Bahrain. "They give us a motor pool where they put the whole battalion," he says. "It was just a big round shed. We built an office out of the plywood packing crates we shipped our tools in. We were heating with kerosene that we're buying downtown, while we're messin' with diesel fuel and gasoline for the trucks. There was no ventilation. So therefore we was breathing that stuff. Then about once a week the Saudis would come through and fog the area for insects. With what, we don't know, but it just covered everything."

"It just came down and hung inside those plastic-covered sheds," adds Jerry's wife, Connie. "The Saudis had no regulations like we do in America."

"There was no prior notice," says Jerry. "You'd hear the trucks start up out there, and here they'd come about forty miles an hour, foggin' all over everything.

"Well, in April, four months after I came, I was sittin' doing paperwork when they come through and fogged one day. The other guy that was helping me, he had gone up to the battalion office, which was an enclosed office at the end of the building. When he came back, I told him, 'You need to take me to the dispensary.' I was getting sick to my stomach, light-headed. My mouth was numb around my lips, my arms was tinglin', my chest was hurtin'. So they took me to the dispensary."

Because Jerry was over forty and overweight, the dispensary doctor treated him for a heart attack. But they could find nothing wrong with him. After four days, he was discharged to go back to work.

"I was feeling better," he says. "I had had IVs, oxygen, and clean air — the ICU unit had its own air filter. I went back to work the next day. We had a company meeting, so I had to go over to the company area, which was about a mile and a half away. While I was gone they come through and fogged. Well, I come back there, and I go in, and I get all my reports ready to turn in, and I'm sittin' there about ten minutes, and I start the same thing. The numbness, chest pains, tingling, and everything. So I tell this guy, 'Let's go again . . .'"

Back in the dispensary, a doctor Jerry hadn't seen before decided to treat him as though he had been a victim of a nerve-agent attack. "He gave me a little white pill and put me on oxygen. I felt better." But before he was discharged, Jerry ran into his original doctor. "He saw the paperwork, laughed, threw it away, and said, 'We're gonna send you outta here and get a stress test.' So they sent me to Germany that night."

All of which enrages Connie Phillips. She's tall, taller than Jerry, blond, strong, formidable. "The papers to treat him for a nerve attack were destroyed," she says. "That's a felony. That's a serious violation of the law. That's a federal document that's part of his legal record. An employee of the government destroyed a federal medical record."

"What was the little white pill?" I ask.

"We don't know," Jerry says. "We don't know if it was pyridostigmine bromide, or what."

"They didn't put the information in his chart," Connie says. "It's destroyed."

Pyridostigmine bromide is a drug that blocks the body's uptake of nerve gas. During the Gulf War, it was given to troops in case of chemical attack. It was up to each commanding officer to order his soldiers to take the pills — every eight hours for up to seven days — when an attack was thought to be imminent. It's likely that the great majority of ground personnel took at least one dose, and probably all twenty-one tablets given them. And there are reports that some troops took repeated rounds of the drug.

Pyridostigmine has been used for decades in patients with myasthenia gravis, a chronic disease marked by extreme fatigue and weakness of muscles, but it has never been approved for general use. The Department of Defense acquired it under a special waiver from the Food and Drug Administration, with the intent of researching the drug, then giving it to personnel with their informed consent. But the soldiers weren't warned that it has side effects, such as memory loss and breathing problems, and the DOD's research ignored key groups — like women — and didn't address the effect of the drug in combination with other exposures — pesticides, for example. These discrepancies have prompted Jay Rockefeller, the outgoing chairman of the Senate Veterans Affairs Committee, to list pyridostigmine as a possible cause of Gulf War syndrome. "The Pentagon had no proof that the drugs and vaccines were safe or effective," he declares.

Jerry Phillips wonders if pyridostigmine bromide, along with the inoculations he received before going to the Gulf, the contents of which were never disclosed to him, and his exposure to Saudi pesticides, also never identified, induced his illness. He wonders whether these combinations of exposures ruined something in his body. After all, this is a guy who used to think WD-40 would make good perfume, and now chemicals were making him sick. The Pentagon might contend that there is no such thing as Gulf War syndrome, but the Phillipses have no doubt at all. Except that's not how they and other sick vets refer to their illness.

"Among the families we call it chemical AIDS," says Connie.

"But don't tell anybody out there that you've got chemical AIDS," says Jerry. "You'll be sittin' there talkin', and then you'll be sittin' there by yourself. What happened? Everybody go to the bathroom at once?"

By April Jerry was back in the States for good. By May, having endured a chaotic hegira from military base to military base, hospital to hospital, diagnosis to diagnosis, he was back home in Oklahoma. And in bad shape.

"He had a month off, and all he did was sleep," says Connie. "I'd leave in the morning for work, he'd be on the couch goin' to sleep. I'd come home, he'd wake up for a few minutes. I'd go to school, he'd go back to sleep. I'd come home later at night, wake him up, and he'd go to bed.

"After he started goin' back to work . . . I figured by this time he should've rested up . . . he'd come in from work, lie on the couch, sleep — same thing. On the weekends he'd sleep from the time he got off work to the time he went to work on Monday morning. Just constantly."

And this lifelong mechanic found he could no longer tolerate the solvents, the paint, the gasoline, the very materials that had never bothered him before. Still, he continued to work, until he was pushed over the edge. Recalls Connie, "We went out and played volleyball one day. It was an indoor court, and there was a weight machine in the corner. There was a guy in there that was using some lacquer thinner to clean the weight machine. Well, Jerry gets about the color of these white walls, and I seen him grab his chest, and he goes outside to get some air. Then he comes back in, says, 'I'm doin' it again.' So I load him up and take him to the hospital."

Another round of mad dashes from base hospital to base hospital, and from diagnosis to diagnosis. Finally Jerry found himself being driven to the office of an allergist in Oklahoma City. "We go in the building, and they're putting down new carpet downstairs," Connie says. "We go upstairs, and Jerry's just beet red. The doctor comes in, takes one look at Jerry, and says, 'I can tell you what's wrong before you tell me anything: you're chemically sensitive.' Then Jerry told him all his symptoms. The doc said probably the reason that Jerry reacted quicker than some of the other vets was that he served three tours in Vietnam and was exposed to Agent Orange. Then he said — and this was the first time anybody had ever explained this to us — 'Your body is like a cup. It can hold only so much. You were already filled to the brim with Agent Orange, and you could not tolerate any more.' He said, 'I can't do anything for you, but I know somebody who can.' And he referred us down here to Dr. Rea."

A clattering in the hall outside. The door springs open, followed by Betty Zuspann pushing Gary in his wheelchair. And Bill Rea.

Rea pats Gary on the back and shakes his head. "How can people deny chemical sensitivity exists?" he says to me. "We've treated about ninety Gulf War veterans here, and we're treating some in England. It's clear they have chemical sensitivity." He nods to Jerry and closes the door behind him.

"He's something," Jerry says. "I came to see him one time, and I had gained some weight. He said, 'Damn, you've blimped up!'"

"We're doing what Dr. Rea tells us to do," says Connie. "We've seen how it can work."

"I have good days and bad days," Jerry says. "The town we live in — to the north of us there's an oil refinery, to the south of us there's a feed mill, and to the west of us there's a tire plant."

"So we have to put up with something all the time," Connie says. "But we've built a safe room. Built a sauna. We have all the exercise equipment you could ever want. People gave it to us. Friends, neighbors."

As Jerry leaves to be examined, he hands me his card. It announces, above his name and phone number, in large, black letters:

P.O.V.A.

Pissed Off Veterans of America.

Jerry Phillips's case is distressing enough. Gary Zuspann's is even worse. Just now, however, he is feeling a little better. He wasn't doing too bad when he and Betty left their little town of Hewitt, down near Waco, a couple of hours south on Interstate 35, but when they drove into Dallas he relapsed. "Just as we got into all this construction, he started vomiting his guts up," Betty says. "He was pale and clammy, and I couldn't figure it out. Is he having an asthma attack? An allergic reaction? What should I do? It was rush-hour traffic, and I was stuck.

There's a car in front of me, to the side of me, and there's a wall over here. I can't pull over to a curb, 'cause there is no curb, they're doin' this construction."

"This is definitely a bad day," Gary says.

But now, sniffing oxygen, breathing the filtered air of the center, he's coming around.

"Well, I was in the navy," he begins in a thin, soft voice. He talks slowly and haltingly, with long pauses. "We sailed December first, 1990. I was thirty then. I was on a helicopter carrier, the *New Orleans*. We toted marines over there, but it was mostly for helicopters. Our first stop was the Philippines; we were there for Christmas and New Year's Day. Then ended up on spot, wherever that spot was, January fifteenth or sixteenth. Whenever the war started, we were where we were supposed to be."

"They were sailing off the coast of Kuwait," Betty clarifies. She does a lot of that. "Gary has a lot of brain damage. Sometimes he won't remember what you say, and you have to repeat it."

"I was a cook," Gary goes on. "In charge of getting meals out to officers, pilots, marines, navy people. We worked anywhere from twelve- to eighteen-hour jobs." He pauses for a moment. "We went up and down the coast. I can't even tell you how many times. We had a SCUD attack."

"I followed the ship's history," Betty says. She's as small and thick as Gary is long and tall. Brown, stringy hair, a blunt oval face, eyes that disappear when she smiles. She's a firecracker, a firebrand. She talks a mile a minute. ("She's a pit bull, ain't she?" Gary says, admiringly.)

"It's amazing what that ship did," Betty says. "They volunteered to go in and chart a map through minefields for other ships. Gary's ship carried the first Americans to reach the Kuwaitis with water and food. They charted the Sacamea oil fields, which were on fire. The slick was there, the wells were on fire out in the water — they charted through that. They charted all the way to Kuwait City, through mines, so that other ships could come in and off-load their marines. They did a lot of their operations coming in and out of those oil fields that were on fire. I talked to marine helicopter pilots who couldn't even find the ship, the smoke was so thick. They had to come in from instruments, get talked in to the ship."

"The air conditioning didn't work very well," says Gary. "The ship takes the air from the outside and recirculates it through the system like a fan does. What's outside comes inside."

"How the ship wasn't blown up I don't know," Betty says.

By February, two and a half weeks after shipping out, Gary reported to sick bay with burning eyes, severe headaches, difficulty swallowing. He took some analgesics and went back to work. "I had problems," he says, "but my mind-set was that it may not have been a very important job but I had responsibilities. I had people under me. I had people over me that would be yelling at me if my job wasn't accomplished. So a headache or sore throat or being uncomfortable or being hot never entered the picture. I figured I wasn't gonna be a whiner. I got a job to do."

Then conditions grew worse. While the *New Orleans* was sailing in and out of the oil fields, the ship's ventilation system broke down. Now the smoke from the oil fires, the reek from the oil slicks, and all the rest of the accumulated gases and odors of shipboard life simply stayed aboard. "And they ingested oil from the water in the Gulf," says Betty. "The ship drank and cooked in this oil. 'Cause they had no bottled water like the troops on land did, they had to drink what was in the oil spill."

Eventually the ship sailed into a Saudi port to be fitted with diesel generators to power the ventilation system and other onboard needs. "So Saudi diesel fuel, which had lead in it and all this other stuff, permeated every recess in the ship," Betty says. "It had nowhere to go."

Gary finally became too sick to carry on. "I left the ship around the end of July, first part of August, I don't remember. . . ."

"August nineteenth," Betty says softly. "When he got off the plane in San Diego, he was gray. He looked like a prisoner of war. He weighed probably a hundred and thirty pounds, down from one seventy five. His eyes were blue — the whites were a pale blue. And when I kissed him, it was like kissing metal. I don't know how else to describe it. Like leaning up against a piece of old lead or steel and kissin' it. I knew something was weird."

Today, as they have for the past three and a half years, Gary and Betty Zuspann live in a prefab structure perched on cinder blocks a foot off the ground in the yard behind his parents' house in Hewitt. It looks like a large tool shed, about 14 feet by 20 feet. You'd never guess anyone lived here — until you got close to the front door. Some fifteen large canisters of oxygen lean against a small porch. On the door itself a sign:

CAUTION
Strong Chemicals Can Be Life-Threatening
to Resident.

In the window to the right of the door, more signs:

CAUTION
Oxygen in use.
No Smoking. No Open Flames. No Matches. No Candles.

CAUTION
A Very Chemically Sensitive, Allergic Person Lives
Here. Do Not Come Into The House If You're Wearing
Perfume, Hair Spray, Deodorant, Dry-Cleaned Clothes.

NO SMOKING ON PREMISES
Do Not Even Knock If You Have Worked In Or Around
Strong Chemicals In The Last 24 Hours, Pesticides,
Herbicides, Formaldehydes, Petrochemicals,
Paint Thinner, Etc.

Betty meets me on the porch, quickly closing the door behind her. "He's sleeping," she says, then invites me inside. I
step into another world. This is the Zuspanns' fortress against
the environment. Their bunker from which to do battle. Their
safe haven where they can survive.

The shed is partitioned into three small rooms. The middle
room, where we stand, contains a gray metal cabinet full of
medical supplies, a huge, noisy air-filtration device, Gary's
wheelchair, a large TV with its backside jutting into the room,
and not much else. Air whooshes through the filter, like a gust-
ing gale wind. The floor is shiny gray linoleum, the walls milky-
white paneling. Aluminum foil blocks the windows. Overhead
fluorescent bulbs bathe the sterile space in an eerie glow.

To the left, through a hardwood door, the kitchen. That is,
the kitchen/laundry room/living room/reading room/office.
"Betty's Room, we call it," she says. It contains a stove, refrigera-
tor, freezer, washer, dryer, a chair, a table crowded with computer, printer, phone, water distiller, and Betty's array of snack
foods: potato chips, Rice Krispies, lemonade — all those things
she would never, ever, serve to Gary. ("There's ten, twelve foods
he can have, and that's about it," she says.) No foil blocks the
window in here. The clear glass offers a look outside to a sunny,
hot August Texas morning. Betty does a lot of her living in this
cluttered room.

Quickly we leave the kitchen behind and return to the
middle room. Lately Gary has been suffering sleep apnea. He's
hooked up to a device that beeps when he stops breathing.
Close the door to the kitchen and you can't hear it. Betty wants
to hear it. So we talk — shout at each other, really — standing

up (there's no place to sit except for the wheelchair), with the air filter roaring, the fluorescent lights humming. She points to the bedroom where Gary sleeps.

"All that's in there is his bed and another purifier and a light and IV pole and a fan," she says. "His bathroom's on the other side. There are speakers for the TV in there that were outgassed for a while. He stays in there most of the time. There's just too many things to make him sick in the other part of the house. And when I take him outside he gets really sick."

She points through the bedroom to Gary's parents' house. "They have a big walk-in closet — that's what they fixed for Gary after he got out of Walter Reed Hospital in Houston. We put up sheets of heavy-duty insulation, totally covered the walls. That's what he lived in for a year until we could get this done.

"I don't know what I'd do without them. Anybody who comes over, they give 'em the rules: no cologne, none of that stuff. But we don't allow a lot of people in here. You're the first person other than family who's been in here to see Gary in a *year*."

Something in my expression stops Betty short. She looks up at me with tears rolling down her cheeks. "Remember the vows? It's called richer or poorer, sickness or health. I'm just glad he's alive. I have friends whose husbands have been buried with the American flag on them. I don't want that feeling at all. I'm very lucky in having him alive. And I'll take him any way I can get him. But we'll get good. He'll get past this stage. He'll — "

Beep! Beep! Beep! The apnea alert. Betty stops talking midsentence and rushes into the bedroom.

Gary's post-Gulf experience was much like Jerry Phillips's, only worse. Similar moving from hospital to hospital and diagnosis to diagnosis, similar frustration, similar growing mistrust of the medical care provided him. But Gary was sicker than Jerry, gravely sick, close-to-death sick, a tougher nut to crack. He was the least desirable of patients — riddled with problems and complaints, responding to no conventional tests or treatments, a sink hole of time and effort for any doc, not to mention overworked, underpaid army physicians who doubted the reality of Gulf War syndrome in the first place. He encountered particular ill will. According to Betty, one of his doctors at Walter Reed Hospital in Houston was an AIDS researcher who was pulled off that disease and given the growing hordes of Persian Gulfers to look after. "She yelled at him every day. She'd lean over his bed and shout, 'Just when are you gonna decide to get out of this damn bed and get up and go home and get you a damn job? Do you realize that you're taking up one of my AIDS patient's beds? He's a lot sicker than you are, and he's gonna have to stay in a hotel . . .'"

Often the diagnosis was depression. And the prescription, Prozac. Betty Zuspann will have none of that.

"When you go to the Veterans Administration to be seen by a medical doctor, the minute they know you're a Persian Gulfer they automatically send you to Psych. Then if they give a diagnosis of psychiatric depression or posttraumatic stress disorder, that is the only thing they have to treat you for. If you accept that diagnosis without appealing, and accept that compensation, then if you come back this month or next month, and another doc says, 'You have a collapsed valve in your heart and it's because of toxic chemicals,' the VA can come back with, 'No, no, that didn't happen in the Gulf. That had to have happened in the last month or two.'

"So what's really goin' on here? You go to the VA or DOD, and the doc says, 'You're stressed.' Or, 'There's nothing wrong with you. Why don't you go home, take some Valium or Prozac?' Then you go to a civilian doctor, and they do a brain scan and echocardiogram and find you got an enlarged heart and brain damage. The civilian guy says, 'You've been exposed to toxic chemicals.' The VA guy says, 'You're depressed.' What's goin' on here?"

So, what *is* going on here? It's a hard question to answer.

"The Persian Gulf War was an experience of unprecedented stress for our military and their families." (So states the *Journal of the American Medical Association* [*JAMA*] in a lengthy report of a Gulf War investigation conducted by the National Institutes of Health.) The onset of the war was quick, the mobilization of troops rapid. It was public knowledge that Iraq had stockpiles of chemical and biological weapons, and it was likely that personnel would be exposed to chemical attacks at the least, biological attacks at the worst. Some fifty thousand casualities were expected should the conflict result in a ground war. And because of the need for secrecy, troops knew little in advance about their destination and prospects. All that caused stress and anxiety.

All troops received vaccinations and other medications to protect against what might await them. And what awaited them was long hours working and living in unsanitary conditions among flies, snakes, spiders, and scorpions, while being exposed to chemical contaminants from oil fires, the burning of feces and trash, fuels and solvents. All in a climate marked by extreme temperatures and the constant presence of ultra-fine sand and dust.

In particular, troops were exposed to:

- Petroleum. Besides the use of petroleum for fuel, petroleum (kerosene, diesel, and leaded gasoline) was used for heating, and petroleum products including diesel fuels were used to keep down sand and dust. And beginning in late February of 1991, military personnel in Kuwait and eastern Saudi Arabia were exposed to oil-well fires.
- Sand and dust. Respiratory problems were reported in al-

most one-third of those who served in the Gulf. Ultra-fine sand embedded in the lungs might be the reason why.

- Pesticides. The use of pesticides in the Gulf was unrestricted and widespread. In addition to institutionalized applications for insect control, individual troops sprayed pesticides on their uniforms and rubbed them on their skin. Saudis also widely applied pesticides. No one knows which ones. No one knows the consequences of exposure.
- Biological and chemical weapons. Whether or not, and to what extent, troops were exposed to chemical and biological agents remains controversial. "Many veterans report that exposures occurred. There were numerous sightings of dead animals. The Czechs reported detection of both sarin and mustard gas in separate incidents," reports *JAMA*. Some vets insisted that thousands of Iraqis inadvertently killed by chemical or biological weapons were buried in mass graves — what they called Operation Desert Sword. "And there were . . . repeated stories of whole herds of camels and goats that had apparently just dropped dead in place and were mysteriously untouched by flies."

For years defense officials reported no evidence of such exposures. But in the spring of 1996 the Pentagon admitted that three hundred to four hundred U.S. troops may have been exposed to chemical weapons — including the deadly nerve agent sarin — due to the destruction of an Iraqi ammunition depot. In the fall the figure was revised to more than five thousand soldiers. The disclosures confirmed long-held suspicions but also raised eyebrows. "I don't know how the Defense Department keeps denying that hundreds of thousands of troops were exposed," stated a former aide to Senator Riegle, James Tuite III, now director of the Gulf War Research Foundation. "They say five thousand now. They will be up to twenty thousand soon." (Sure enough, in October of 1996 the Pentagon revised the figure to at least twenty thousand.)

- Depleted uranium. Another potential problem. Radio-activity from uranium-tipped shells was ostensibly below acceptable standards, but no one knows its impact.
- Pyridostigmine bromide. Past experience prescribing py-ridostigmine for myasthenia gravis suggests that it causes no long-term difficulties. But up to half of treated troops reported side effects from the drug. Another mystery area.
- Vaccines. Persian Gulfers were vaccinated against common infectious diseases as well as against two agents of bio-logical warfare, anthrax and botulism toxin. While the infectious-disease vaccines are routinely given to military personnel and civilians, vaccines against anthrax and botu-lism are less widespread. Still, they've been given to thou-sands of people with no long-term problems. Yet reports persist of severe reactions to the inoculations. One navy nurse claims that over half of the people to whom she gave anthrax vaccines reacted adversely, with "huge" swellings and high fever.

  Some people also contend that vaccines other than standard preparations approved by the Food and Drug Ad-ministration were given to Persian Gulfers. Experimental drugs, for example. Patricia Axelrod of Takoma Park, Maryland, who has been studying Desert Storm com-plaints with a $60,000 grant from the John D. and Cather-ine T. MacArthur Foundation contends that the military "does not want it known that Desert Storm was a living laboratory. Americans were exposed to toxic environmen-tal circumstances, including chemical- and biological-warfare agents. They have used these people as guinea pigs . . ."

No matter the truth of these allegations, all agree that what isn't known, and needs to be investigated, is the effect of combinations of exposures. Any one exposure may or may not be dangerous in itself, but could they prove especially harmful together? What is the synergistic effect of the variety of exposures experienced by troops during the Persian Gulf War?

If much that happened during the war remains obscure and troubling for ailing vets, in its own way the aftermath has been every bit as rough. All the more so because many vets feel that they have been treated shabbily by the VA and DOD, the very institutions that are supposed to be on their side. The complaints mirror those of the Zuspanns and Phillipses:

• **Superficial treatment.** Carol Picou, a nurse from Universal City, Texas, served in the Gulf and now suffers from Gulf War syndrome. She contends that vets are given only cursory examinations. "They ask you what's wrong, draw some blood, send for chest X rays, and that's it. If you have rashes, they may send you for a dermatology appointment, which takes three to six months."

Betty Zuspann claims that one of Gary's doctors said to him, "It's a shame you don't have AIDS, 'cause then I could give you all the help you could stand. But because you're a Persian Gulf vet, I can only test you. I can't treat you."

"'Why?'" I asked.

"'Because Washington won't let us . . .'"

• **Missing medical records.** Jerry Phillips's complaint that records of his treatment for a possible nerve-gas attack were destroyed resembles the experience of many vets. Dean Lundholm, a Santa Cruz, California, reservist who served as a prisoner-of-war guard, says he spent several days unconscious in the hospital while in the Gulf, but that "now all files pertaining to that seem to have disappeared." Another veteran claims that medical records for his entire unit are missing. Some claim they saw medical records being burned and that some of their test results have been classified.

According to Betty Zuspann, when Gary was at Walter Reed Hospital in Washington, D.C., "one of the nurses noticed that his gums were bleeding. She put it in her chart, and they made her take it out. She *told* me they made her take it out."

And at the VA hospital in Houston, when Gary received a second opinion from a non-military doctor, "He wrote in Gary's chart — I saw it 'cause I used to go down and read Gary's chart — 'Take him to Methodist Hospital because the VA equipment is not adequate.' Well, that was torn out of the chart at a later date."

• **"Psychological conditions."** Often the crux of veterans' complaints is the old bugaboo of civilian MCS-ers: being told that the problem is all in their heads.

"Most of our soldiers are being referred to psych wards," if they get referrals at all, says Carol Picou. "Our stress is coming from the fact that we're sick, and we can't get anybody to help us."

Connie Phillips agrees: "You're afraid to have any testing from the VA, because they can always somehow make it look like it's psychiatric depression."

Betty Zuspann thinks she understands why. "They're afraid to admit there's a problem. It's easier just to say that the problem is not real, just diagnose these vets with depression, than to say, 'My judgment and education isn't what it should be. Maybe I shoulda picked up the phone and called another doctor for an opinion.' If they recognize these vets' disease, they're gonna have to give them health care. And it's cheaper to bury them than it is to give them care."

• **Careless, unfeeling treatment.** "When they transferred Gary to the VA in Houston," Betty says, "I fought with them from the moment he went in there to bring in an environmental physician that was experienced in chemical sensitivities and serious chemical allergies. And they refused. The chief of staff down there kept trying to convince me that he was just depressed. I mean, I was constantly having to fight to get him to bring in any kind of specialist at all.

"We used to get into screaming matches. 'Well, what are you gonna do if a specialist comes down here and says he's depressed?' And I'd come back with, 'Then he's depressed. We'll treat it. But what are you gonna do if he's chemically sensitive? Are you gonna have enough guts to put that in a chart? I don't trust y'all as far as I can throw you.'

"Meanwhile, there was a bathroom across the hall from Gary's room and they put a deodorizer in there and it leaked. He got catatonic. It was like he was in a coma or something. His eyes were open, but he couldn't respond.

"'Are you happy now?' I told them. 'I *demand* a specialist! I'm gonna bring in Ted Koppel and anybody else I can get down here, and I'll get *him* to get us a specialist.'

"So I wrote down the names of five specialists on a list. Dr. Rea, Doris Rapp . . . and they marked out everybody but Claudia Miller. 'Cause she's from the University of Texas in San Antonio. They didn't know who Claudia Miller was, but they're kinda connected with UT. So Dr. Miller came, and she said he definitely had had exposures. Just pesticide spraying alone was enough to have an effect. It was the first time a doctor had said that. She was shocked when she found out that they did pesticide spraying in the berthing areas where sailors sleep on ships. They'd spray once a week, and there's no ventilation down there.

"She came back from San Antonio a couple more times, to try to educate them and give classes. A sign was placed on Gary's door that said, 'Chemically Sensitive Patient. No One Allowed Wearing Cologne, etc. . . .'

"But the doctors there, they don't care. They have no scruples or morals or nothing. They get a check, they do what they're told, and they don't do what's right. I was there for three months. I slept there. I was there twenty-four hours a day.

I saw things in there that'd shut a hospital down and put the people in jail. Soldiers are equipment, like a tank or gun. And when they're broken they're no use anymore — that's the attitude. They could care less if they live or die."

It's this kind of mistreatment that has prompted Betty to become a link in the network of Gulf War veteran groups. Her post, one of eight in Texas and of some seventy-five nationwide and in the United Kingdom and Canada, is called the Desert Storm Veterans Coalition. When you call her 800 number, you get this message, delivered in as calm a voice as I've ever heard from Betty:

"Persian Gulf Hotline, where veterans are helping each other. Thousands of Persian Gulf soldiers who served in the Gulf and their families are ill, as a result of that service. Veterans organizations like ours are trying to get information out to these soldiers and their families. If you'll send for a request by leaving your name, your complete address, and, if you want to, your phone number, we'll get a packet out to you as soon as possible."

That's the kind of thing she does at the computer in "Betty's Room." And she has a small storage room down the block where she keeps her arsenal of newspaper and magazine articles, congressional reports, military documents, and other records of the plight of Persian Gulfers. (She can go there, however, only when she arranges for someone to stay in the shed with Gary.) Betty has testified before Congress, giving that staid body a dose of her Texas grit. She has spoken at medical conferences, and she has encountered firsthand what Desert Storm vets experienced routinely.

"A lot of the guys were shipping me some of their stuff to give to Congress for them to research," she recalls. "I opened what I thought was a grid map that a soldier had pulled out of an Iraqi bunker. It had been sealed since it came out of the theater. I pulled open this plastic sack that had foil wrapped around it, and got *mustard-gassed!*

"My hands were burning, my mouth was burning, my throat, my esophagus — I still got damage in my esophagus. I ran to the sink and washed my hands, and the more I washed them, the more they burned.

"They had to rush me to the emergency room in an ambulance. I was gagging like you want to throw up, dry heavin' and you can't quit. The stupid doctor didn't believe that I had been exposed to some kind of gas or toxic chemicals. He just laughed. He wrote on my chart that I hyperventilated.

"That map got sent to Lawrence Livermore labs, and everybody who's handled it has gotten sick. They said it was dusty mustard. They said there was something else on the map too, but they couldn't figure out what it was. So they sent it somewhere else. We haven't heard about that."

The experience deepened her conviction that GWS, whatever it is, is being spread from the returning vets to their families. Probably from exposure to the stuff they brought back from the Gulf — which many vets and their families suspect was contaminated not only with chemicals, but with agents of biological warfare. As far as Betty is concerned, Gulf War syndrome is contagious.

"What starts with the wives is these awful headaches. They are *horrible*. I've had migraines before but I've never had headaches like that in my life. But the pain in the back of the neck is the worst. Kinda like somebody's pushin' a book down on your head, or an anvil. Then you think your eyes are goin' bad. That's the kind of symptoms you're gonna see in the wives, and the children who was born before the war, when they brought all the duffel bags and everything back. You're gonna find that even nurses that have taken care of these soldiers are sick.

"Connie Phillips and I have been on antibiotics for two, three years now, 'cause we've been working so closely with vets. I have good days and bad days. I can go to one of these meetings where there's a lot of these sick vets, and I'm in bed for almost a week. I don't know what they're giving me, but as long as I take my antibiotics I do really good.

"Don't look like that," she tells me. "It only happens to anybody who's been around them for any real length of time. Dr. Rea will tell you that. You've just been around a little bit."

But Connie and Jerry Phillips are not so reassuring. Maybe because they have a two-year-old grandson, the child of a son who also was in the Gulf and also became ill, who was born with a shortage of red blood cells — an abnormality they blame on GWS. In their minds, there's no doubt that this illness is contagious.

"It's transmittable," Jerry says.

"Transmitted by saliva and sweat," adds Connie.

"They say it can even be transmitted by shaking hands."

Connie levels a glance at me. "You're a brave man."

Betty emerges from the darkened bedroom. It was a false alarm. No apnea this time — Gary's awake. Would I like to come in and say hello?

I pull off my shoes and put on cotton hospital-style booties. Betty rolls in the wheelchair for me. And there propped up on pillows in an imitation brass bed, oxygen line running into his nose, lies Reserve Navy Petty Officer Third Class Gary Zuspann.

"It's amazing what an old tool shed can look like, ain't it?" he says in his thin, soft voice. "It's home for now."

He laboriously rearranges himself, pushes up higher on his pillows. He's still pale, but less peaked than in Dallas. "I haven't been letting very many people over — "

"You're lucky," Betty says to me. "Not very many people get to come in here." She hovers over Gary like a mother over a child, props up his pillows, completes his slow sentences, fills in the gaps during pauses.

" — because I didn't want to expose anybody to anything," he continues. "We still don't know what all's goin' on. I have a little nephew I haven't seen in a long, long time."

"Three years!" says Betty.

"I'm afraid I might get him sick. It's kinda difficult."

A TV remote control, portable phone, and radio sit by the side of the bed. A metal fan pushes air around. The large TV in the middle room is visible through a glass panel. The door to the bathroom is closed behind us. Foil blocks the window. Home, Sweet Home.

"I guess in a lot of ways I'm a very lucky man," Gary says. "Because a lot of people don't think it's real. Reason why I'm lucky is . . . I finally got a doc who didn't tell me it was all in my head and go out and get a job . . .

"I have a new computer comin'," Gary says. "That's something the VA has finally approved after a couple of years. I got a new counselor, and he's real ballsy. So he's tryin' to get stuff done that I hadn't been able to get done before. They're supposed to pick it up sometime this week. Then they're gonna build a hood for it, where all the vapors and everything go up into an air purifier."

"Suck out whatever it has to suck out," says Betty.

"It'll be glassed off and everything," Gary says. "I'll be able to open it and put in CDs and get on the Internet and all that neat stuff. I'm really lookin' forward to that.

"We're gonna have an electrician in and put an electrical box on that side," he says to Betty.

"Uh-huh, we'll get that done," she says.

"And a phone line over there, too."

"Uh-huh, we'll get that done. You'll be *all* hooked up. You can talk to everybody on the Internet then."

"Yeah, I reckon. I don't know how expensive it'll be . . ."

"You don't worry about that. Jerry's got his computer now. Y'all can talk to each other. They have a Persian Gulf bulletin board on there, all the sick vets talkin' to each other."

"Why do you have the windows blocked off?" I ask.

"Well, the glass that they put into this building isn't double-pane glass," Gary explains. "They were the windows that came with the building. It's not a real tight seal. The foil keeps some of the smells out. And it insulates a little bit more."

"When we get in a new house, though . . ." Betty says.

"It'll be done right."

"I'm glad the foil is up there," she says. "'Cause when he gets a real bad headache, these throbbing, throbbing head-aches, it has to be totally dark in here. It's not that often. Usu-ally from somethin' I've done — brought somethin' in, given him somethin', and he reacts to it. Usually because of some stupid reason.

"Like these channel changers." She grabs the TV remote. "We fought Gary about the channel changers, me and Dr. Rea both did. Thought he might react to the plastic. There was a big rah-rah fight about the channel changers. He'd say, 'You've taken everything else away from me, at least I can have my channel changer!'"

Gary laughs. It's the first time I've seen him laugh. His face absolutely lights up, a full, delighted grin, like a child.

"Finally Dr. Rea said, '*Stick 'em in there!* He's gonna gripe about 'em all the time, it's gonna upset him that much, stick 'em in there.' That was about two years ago, I remember that battle.

"Then we ended up with three channel changers. Not two, not one, but *three!* One for the TV, one for the music, one for the videos. I told Dr. Rea, 'Well, he's up to three channel changers.'

"He said, 'I told him he can only have one.'

"I said, 'I'm not fightin' him over it. You tell him he can't have three.'"

So it goes. Days blur into nights for the Zuspanns. An elabo-rate holding action — waiting out his illness, living Bill Rea's dictum of "Avoidance, Avoidance, Avoidance" to the max, Gary eating his limited menu of organic foods, sticking to a rotation diet, wondering what's in store. Trying to make plans ("Pretty soon you'll have to make out your list of what you want for Christmas," Betty says. "How 'bout a new house? Wouldn't that work?") but unable to make plans. Trying to keep spirits high.

"You got two choices," Gary says. "You can either roll over and play dead, or you can put up one hell of a fight until the end. I don't want to make it too easy on 'em."

"Do you think about dying?" I ask.

"I try not to. I guess if I was still at a hundred and twenty-nine pounds, and I was still in a wheelchair all the time . . . if I was still in the situation I was in five years ago and not gettin' better but worse. . . . Even though I'm in a limiting situation, it doesn't mean it's over. You never know how strong you are until you're put into a situation where you're tested."

"Find out what you're made of," Betty says.

"I think that things are slowly changing anyway. I think people are becoming more cautious of the environment anyway. Least that's the sense I'm getting from watching TV."

"But they don't think of themselves as being in the environment," Betty says, "We've had a lot of discussions about that, a lot of *heated* discussions," she tells me.

"I understand that," Gary says. "But I guess what I'm saying is that we got organic foods that are now becoming more popular. It's the in thing to eat organic. It's the in thing to wear cotton clothes. It's the in thing not to live in the city, but live away from the city where the air is cleaner. I just think slowly things are startin' to turn around. I see some exciting getting-back-to-basics in the next century . . ."

On April 17, 1996, the *New York Times* ran this headline: "Chemical Mix May Be Cause of Illnesses in Gulf War." Researchers at Duke University and the University of Texas

Southwestern Medical Center in Dallas finally had done the obvious: they tested the effect of exposure to combinations of common chemicals. Their "guinea pigs" were chickens, the animals usually preferred for such studies because they react much as humans do (since they have only two legs, they fall over like people should they become disoriented), and the chemicals they tested were ones actually used in the Gulf. When the team gave the chickens single doses of one chemical or another, they could detect no signs of illness. But when they combined them, things started to happen.

The chemicals they used were pyridostigmine, the ubiquitous anti–nerve gas tablets, and the pesticides DEET and permethrin. DEET is an insect repellent used by the military since 1946, and by the general public since 1957. It's applied directly to the skin. Permethrin, an insecticide, is also applied to the skin.

At first the researchers set out to determine how much of each chemical the animals could stand without becoming ill. The resulting doses were at least three times as much as the soldiers most likely received. This outcome reassured the team that they weren't distorting the Gulf experience. "Even if a person was exposed to one chemical alone at three times the recommended dose, he or she would have remained healthy," says Duke pharmacologist Mohamed Abou-Donia, the head of the research team.

Abou-Donia and his colleagues then gave the chickens combinations of any two of the chemicals. Now results were different. The animals began to show varying degrees of weight loss, diarrhea, shortness of breath, weakness, stumbling, tremors — in other words, Gulf War syndrome–like symptoms. And the chickens exposed to combinations of all three chemicals were worse off, sometimes becoming paralyzed or even dying. Lab tests showed widespread nervous-system damage in the birds.

The inference was inescapable: exposure to a combination

of these chemicals, or ones like them, might have caused Gulf War syndrome.

But why? Why would a combination of exposures cause problems where single exposures didn't? The answer, the researchers found, involves an enzyme in the blood whose job it is to remove foreign chemicals from the body. Called plasma butyrylcholinesterase (BuChE), it acts like a scavenger and culls out foreign invaders such as DEET and permethrin. But there's only so much BuChE in the bloodstream. An exposure to DEET or permethrin alone causes no problems — there's enough BuChE to inactivate any one chemical. Not so with multiple doses — they simply overwhelm the BuChE supply. The result is an accumulation of toxins in the bloodstream that make their way to the brain and nervous system. And the consequence of that is the myriad symptoms experienced by the chickens — and, by extension, the Persian Gulf vets.

But all that ignores pyridostigmine. And here's where things become particularly interesting. When pyridostigmine is added to the mix, the consequences become even worse. Pyridostigmine protects against nerve gas by temporarily shielding the target of the nerve agents, another bloodstream enzyme, called acetylcholine esterase, or AChE, which regulates the nervous system. But AChE and BuChE are similar enzymes, and pyridostigmine doesn't differentiate very well between them. Inadvertently it tends to shield them both, in effect removing both from circulation. Now even less BuChE is available to combat DEET and permethrin. "Pyridostigmine bromide actually pumps more of the other chemicals to the brain," says Abou-Donia. "It magnifies the effects of the other two chemicals by tying up the available BuChE." And if a soldier should happen to be one of the 3 or 4 percent of the population who are born with a faulty form of BuChE, and thus a reduced ability to inactivate chemicals to begin with, the effect of pyridostigmine further diminishing the body's BuChE antichemical capability is even more devastating.

But wait — the story is not over yet. Recall that pyridostigmine's primary task is to temporarily neutralize that other enzyme, AChE. AChE's normal function is to modulate nervous-system activity, in effect dampen down the fire so that our behavior remains on an even keel. But if soldiers took higher-than-recommended doses of pyridostigmine as an added precaution against nerve gas attacks, they may have disrupted that balance. Without AChE to moderate it, the nervous system can become overexcited. The upshot can be tremors, muscle spasms, and other Gulf War syndrome–like symptoms. So at the same time that it was promoting these problems by neutralizing BuChE, pyridostigmine may have been exacerbating the situation by getting rid of AChE. A double-whammy.

Ironically, then, the very measures urged on troops to protect them against danger during the Gulf War may have led to their problems afterward. "The decision to use these chemicals was made to protect soldiers from indigenous diseases in the Gulf," says Abou-Donia. "Without protection, there may have been thousands of deaths. But it appears that, for some veterans, the precautions prevented one set of problems and created another."

Chickens, however, are not human beings. It remains to be seen if this lead pans out with real people. Other recent studies do lend credence to the Duke-Texas effort, though. A Scottish researcher found evidence of nerve damage in ill Persian Gulfers when compared with healthy vets, as did a study based in Israel. Others have found immune-system abnormalities in ailing vets. But more needs to be done. At this writing the Duke-Texas research team is preparing to announce the results of a follow-up study analyzing blood samples from veterans to determine if low enzyme activity is associated with illness. If so, the study would reinforce the notion that multiple chemical exposure knocks out a portion of the body's protective capability. It would be yet another piece of evidence implicating chemicals as the culprit behind Gulf War syndrome.

In January of 1977, in three articles published in *JAMA*, Texas Southwestern researchers further nailed down a causal connection between chemical exposure and Gulf War syndrome. They broke down the illness into three primary syndromes — 'impaired cognition syndrome," characterized by distractibility, difficulty remembering, depression, insomnia, fatigue, confusion, and other problems; "confusion-ataxia syndrome," characterized by problems with thinking and reasoning; and "arthro-myo-neuropathy syndome," characterized by joint and muscle pains, difficulty lifting heavy objects, fatigue, and tingling or numbness in extremities. And all these problems, the researchers concluded, might be the result of wartime exposure to combinations of chemicals such as nerve agents, flea collars, anti–nerve gas pills — that is, pyridostigmine bromide — and insect repellent.

"The findings of our study provide, to our knowledge, the first epidemiologic evidence of associations between environmental risk factors and systematically defined syndromes in Gulf War veterans," the researchers wrote.

In a commentary on the Texas studies, while cautioning that "the link between chemical warfare exposure and disease in Gulf War veterans certainly has not been proven," *JAMA* stated that "the data on symptoms confirm what many physicians caring for Gulf War veterans already know, namely, that the illnesses in these men and women are quite real."

What these studies don't begin to explain, however, are the claims of those who contend that the malady is contagious. But that mystery, too, may start to give up its secrets. The VA has earmarked $2 million for studies of the spouses and children of Gulf vets. It may not be a whopping beginning ("Two million dollars sounds like a lot of money, but you know how the government handles a budget," cautions a Gulf War veterans support group), and vets are notoriously suspicious about military efforts in this area. But it *is* a beginning.

* * *

None of this surprises Gary and Betty Zuspann, or Jerry and Connie Phillips. No surprise to Bill Rea, either. And no surprise to Claudia Miller. She has long suspected chemical involvement in Gulf War syndrome — especially because the illness so closely mirrors MCS. "MCS is very applicable here," she says. "I can think of nothing else that would begin to explain what's going on with the veterans. They have the same kinds of intolerances to chemicals, drugs, and foods that MCS patients do. I think they may be the same thing."

In fact, the symptoms of the two maladies are virtually identical. Below is a chart Miller made up to compare symptoms of Gulf vets to those of MCS sufferers exposed to organophosphates, and to compare both to healthy people — that is, controls. The numbers represent percentage of people complaining.

Symptom	*Vets*	*MCS*	*Controls*
1. Fatigue	76.7	67.6	2.7
2. Joint pain	70	43.2	3.6
3. Tiredness	63.3	62.2	6.3
4. Loss of motivation	53.3	43.2	7.1
5. Muscle aches	50	48.6	1.8
6. Memory difficulties	43.3	56.8	5.4
7. Diarrhea	40	27	0
8. Headache	40	37.8	4.5
9. Abdominal pain	36.7	27	2.7
10. Stiffness	36.7	27	1.8
11. Tingling fingers/toes	33.3	43.2	0.9

12. Concentration difficulties	30	54.1	2.7
13. Frequent urination	30	18.9	0.9
14. Recurrent infections	30	37.8	0
15. Numbness	30	40.5	0.9
16. Weak arms	30	37.8	0
17. Weight gain	30	35.1	14.3
18. Chest pain	26.7	43.2	1.8
19. Muscle cramping	26.7	24.3	2.7
20. Depression	26.7	48.6	6.3
21. Problems focusing eyes	26.7	48.6	4.5
22. Grogginess	26.7	37.8	0
23. Nausea	26.7	18.9	0
24. Weight loss	26.7	21.6	1.8

The results display a pretty close correspondence between MCS and GWS, considering the difference between the genders of the groups. Most of the Gulf vets were men; most of the MCS-ers and controls were women (more about that in a moment).

Moreover, ailing vets experience the same "spreading" phenomenon as do people suffering from MCS. For example, of the first fifty-nine Gulf veterans seen at the Houston VA hospital, 78 percent reported new intolerances to odors of chemicals — in particular, diesel exhaust, solvents, gasoline, tobacco smoke, hair spray and fragrances. Seventy-eight percent reported the onset of food intolerances. Forty percent became intolerant to drugs and medications. Seventy-four percent of those who smoked became intolerant to tobacco. Sixty-six percent of drinkers could no longer drink. Twenty-five percent of coffee drinkers became intolerant to caffeine. And more than three-fourths of them reported the onset of intolerances to two or more of these categories. The similarities between Gulf War syndrome and MCS are arresting.

So why haven't the DOD and VA required that all sick Gulf War vets with these symptoms be screened for MCS? Why haven't the DOD and VA ever released data on the prevalence of these symptoms among Gulf War vets? Why hasn't the DOD issued MCS diagnostic guidelines to all its staff? Why have VA officials specifically instructed local VA doctors *not* to report either the symptoms or diagnosis of MCS? Many Gulf vets might say that, as usual, the Pentagon is trying to put a damper on the problem of Gulf War syndrome — that, as usual, it is not revealing everything it knows.

One may as well ask, however, GWS or no, why isn't MCS widely recognized as a real disease? The answers to all these questions may be obscured in the same murky waters as everything else having to do with this maddening malady. It is simply debilitating, frustrating, and elusive, for those suffering it as well as for those trying to understand it and treat it.

With all that in mind, therefore, the implications of the possibility that multiple chemical sensitivity and Gulf War syndrome are the same multiheaded monster are especially intriguing. While MCS provides a vantage point from which to view the chaos surrounding GWS, it is hardly less messy itself. Seeing GWS in an MCS light does little to clear up the picture — although it may suggest ways of investigating and treating the syndrome. With recent studies such as the Duke-Texas effort, those investigating GWS seem to be doing pretty well on their own. They may not need an MCS handle to help sort things out.

Rather, the greatest benefit may be to reverse the mirror and view MCS in the light of GWS. One of the reasons MCS-ers have traveled such a rocky road in trying to have their malady recognized by the mainstream medical community has been

the makeup of the population that suffers it. MCS is overwhelmingly an affliction of women, and middle-aged women
at that. It has been too easy for some to dismiss the symptoms
of MCS as physical manifestations of the psychological problems of middle-aged females. The reorientation necessitated
by kids leaving the house, the challenge of finding a new role
other than mother and confidante, the challenge of forging a
new, independent identity, all compounded by the impending
onset of menopause.

Well, Gulf War syndrome attracts quite a different constitu-
ency. GWS is overwhelmingly an affliction of men — and
young, fit, active men at that. In GWS you can substitute a
male army vet for a female housewife, and a Saudi motor pool
or oil-well fire in Kuwait for a sick building. And those substi-
tutions are precisely the point. Gulf War syndrome spotlights
the problem in a brand-new guise, a mainstream guise, a *male*
guise, one that may afford it wider acceptance. "There are real
gender biases at work here," says Claudia Miller. "Now you
have Gulf veterans, some of whom were rangers, guys with
black belts in karate. They were healthy when they went over
there. Now they're disabled. They're not middle-aged females.
That makes them more credible in some ways. I think this will
be a real breakthrough for MCS."

Chapter 8

Canaries in the Coal Mine

"THE PEOPLE WHO LIVE in aluminum foil–lined rooms or on top of mountains, like in Wimberley, make very good stories. But they're extreme," Claudia Miller told me in San Antonio. "People can't identify with them. They look like they're crazy because they're living such extreme lives. Yet there are thousands of MCS patients who day to day are just barely coping, trying to work and maintain normal lives."

She's right, of course. And that's the irony of MCS. At the extreme it's such a bizarre malady, this business of being allergic to everything, of escaping the twentieth century by fleeing to remote places or sequestering yourself in specially constructed bunkers. The disease — and the lifestyle it promotes — breeds oddness and eccentricity. Perhaps *attracts* oddness and eccentricity. And so these people — these long-suffering, often miserable people — find themselves objects of derision, the butt of jokes. Or what may be the most stinging rebuke of all: they are simply not believed. As though these people *prefer* to live their lives under siege. As though they get a kick out of constantly treading cautiously through an environment loaded with toxic land mines. As though they lack basic civilized virtues — moral fiber or gumption or tolerance or just plain manners.

Meanwhile, the mass of afflicted people, most of the 15 percent or so of the population that report increased sensitivity to chemicals, quietly go about their business within the mainstream of society. They don't head for the hills or go underground. Rather, they just continue — or *try* to continue — coping day by day. And that means living not only with the runny nose and cough and stinging eyes and rash associated with conventional allergies, but with the chronic headache, the persistent anxiety, the tiresome fatigue, the disruptive brain fog, the deadly depression, or worse, that defines MCS. That means perpetually trying to function when you're not at your best, when you're hardly able to function at all. That means no longer even remembering what it's like to be at your best. And often that means not being able to avoid the source of your habitual irritations, in some cases not even being aware of the source. Rather, just wearily accepting your day-to-day lot in life. These are the people who suffer silently. Thoreau said, "The mass of men lead lives of quiet desperation." In the case of MCS, one might add, "lives of quiet misery."

For all those people, the hard-core MCS community has a message: You're not alone. You're not inherently ill — the environment makes you so. There may be something you can do about your distress, starting with becoming aware of its source.

And for the rest of us, those of us who aren't chemically sensitive, the MCS community has a message as well: You're next!

It used to be a tradition in the coal mines of the eastern United States and elsewhere to place canaries down the shafts before miners themselves ventured inside. The reason had to do with the accumulation of hazardous gases underground. Methane and carbon monoxide are especially dangerous. A mixture of

5 to 15 percent methane in the air can cause violent explosions. And carbon monoxide is poisonous — a whiff can kill you. The canary functioned as a detection device, a living sensor. If the bird continued to chirp, the miners knew that the coast was clear. If the bird fell off its perch and died — better not go down there!

People with MCS consider themselves the human equivalents of canaries in the coal mine. (One MCS-er calls her newsletter *The Singing Canary;* another entitles a recent book *A Canary's Tale.*) Just as the canaries detected dangerous gases, and paid for their trouble, so people with MCS detect dangerous environmental exposures — and pay for their trouble. And just as canaries saved the lives of miners, so MCS-ers might save the health of the rest of us — if we would pay attention. That's the breakdown in the analogy. Coal miners paid attention to the fate of the canaries — crucial, intense, life-or-death attention. We ignore the message posed by people with MCS — or denigrate it, or laugh at it. In effect, what these people are saying is, "Look at us. We are the casualties of our industrial age. Here, but for the grace of God, go you. If conditions don't improve, we are what you will become! Pay attention!" Few do.

Claudia Miller would like to remedy that. In her view, MCS is well worth paying attention to. "Those of us who see chemical sensitivity as an emerging theory for disease see something profoundly different and deeply concerning," she says. Even if there's no consensus as to what's actually at the root of the disease, it's worth paying attention to. What's badly needed, then, is to nail down the cause of MCS once and for all.

The point is that the etiology of MCS *is* testable. "Unlike for cancer or heart disease, cause and effect in MCS can be tested experimentally in humans," Miller says. The effort wouldn't depend on lab rats, or rabbits, or monkeys. No need for cautious translations of the results of animal studies to humans.

This would be examining the real thing with real people. In Miller's view, it must be done, and soon. "What needs to be done now is to demonstrate whether or not chemical sensitivity exists. And the way you do that is blinded challenges in a controlled environment. You have to take the straight road, get away from these arguments that have gone on for forty years, and once and for all determine if this illness can occur in response to low-level challenges. I've thought about this a lot and I don't see any other way."

Al Levin agrees. "The big problem we have is that there's no science. It's all politics. It would be so nice if people just quieted down and said, 'Let's investigate this and find out what's going on.' Because the real enemy is not each other — it's the disease."

In 1993 the National Institute of Environmental Health Sciences described the concept of environmental control unit testing as the "single most important way to develop a reliable clinical approach to the diagnosis and evaluation of chemical sensitivities." But today, in this country, except for Bill Rea's ECU, no such facility exists. And the impact of the Dallas facility in the wider medical community has been negligible. "What goes on in units like Rea's or Randolph's, when he had a unit, is not believed," says Miller. "Physicians who write grants and make decisions haven't been brought into the picture. This testing needs to be done in a university setting."

So why are there no other ECUs? One reason, says Miller, is that the rancor between the mainstream medical camp and the clinical ecology camp has virtually paralyzed the field. "Because of the ongoing debate there's an unwillingness to move forward. I don't even know whom to blame." Another is the sensationalized portrait of MCS promoted by the media. Who wants to pay for an expensive facility to study loonies?

Another reason is that MCS threatens our notion of what constitutes disease and threatens influential blocks of physicians who uphold conventional definitions. "Medical care costs in this nation have risen from 5.3% of gross domestic product in 1960 to 13.9% in 1993, with a dollar value exceeding $1 trillion, nearly $4,000 per person," Miller writes. "The question is, how much does chemical sensitivity contribute to this sum? It's a vexing question that goes against the grain of accepted explanations concerning the origins of illness."

And another reason there is no money for an ECU is the fact that unlike some other diseases — infectious diseases, say, or genetic diseases — MCS by its very nature points an accusing finger at large, important, and influential industries. "MCS hasn't generated private funding like chronic fatigue and other problems have. No drug company wants to fund it as they have done with other research because," Miller says dryly, "drugs don't seem to be appreciated by these patients. And some drug companies are owned by chemical companies. So there's a real lack of resources for looking into this problem."

What she is saying, tactfully, is that chemical and drug industries, which between them spend enormous sums on research, aren't particularly excited at the prospect of designating money for studies of a mysterious, sometimes debilitating illness whose origins may implicate the industries themselves. They're not going to throw big money at something that may cost them bigger money. The result is that for the most part, funds for MCS have simply not been forthcoming. Not from the federal government and not from private sources. Which is a shame, because all that is needed is money. How to construct an environmental control unit is well known, study protocols are in place, facilitators are ready and willing. "Currently, the *only* obstacle to these studies being undertaken is lack of funding," states Miller.

Funding has come through, however, for one promising effort. Not in this country, but in Halifax, Nova Scotia, and not sponsored by any U.S. agency, but by the government of Nova Scotia itself. At Dalhousie University, epidemiologist Michel Joffres is overseeing a large, multifaceted study to try to put to rest some of the confusion surrounding MCS once and for all. The most ambitious leg of this endeavor involves some seven hundred people who in the late 1980s were exposed to an accidental release of ammonia-based chemicals called ammines, which are used to prevent corrosion in boiler systems, and other toxins in a large medical center in the city. Of those seven hundred people, *three hundred* have gone on to develop full-blown MCS — over 40 percent of the whole, an unheard-of percentage.

Since Joffres's team can pinpoint the moment of exposure, they can follow the development of symptoms from a single instant in time, in hundreds of people. It is a rare opportunity. "We can follow the natural history of the illness," he says. "Some people became sick and developed MCS, some people did not. It will be interesting to know why some did and some didn't." And it will be interesting to determine if the medical center accident was the cause. Especially because the Worker's Compensation Board in the area admits that exposure took place, but does not recognize the progression into MCS. Joffres's research may put the lie to such myopia, while providing a profile of the onset of the illness unmatched in any comparably sized group of people. (The Dalhousie Clinical Research Centre is no stranger to MCS. "We are seeing five hundred people with MCS, with another thousand on the waiting list," Joffres says. All these from Nova Scotia alone.)

Besides conducting this large study, Joffres and his team are planning to investigate the effectiveness of provocation-neutralization and vitamin-mineral therapy. To do so, they are building a mini-ECU ("it will be ultra-clean, probably the best in the world") suitable for specific tests. (An ECU for long-term diagnosis and treatment remains a gleam in Joffres's eye. "We don't yet have the money to build that facility.") They are also investigating the utility of SPECT scans, and hope to look into other MCS therapies. "We might also do some monitoring of what happens when people clean up their houses, and compare that to people who do not."

All of this at a respected, mainstream medical facility. "These trials are exactly what are needed," says Joffres. "They will be randomized, double-blinded, placebo-controlled studies. If MCS is to be accepted by the medical community, we have to do it this way."

But he has no illusions that his work will be readily accepted, no matter the results. "I'm under a lot of potential fire," he says. "It's a dangerous business. People are already waiting for a *faux pas*. People are already trying to destroy what we're doing. It's amazing how emotional this issue is. Positively volatile."

That's need number one: determine the cause of multiple chemical sensitivity. Assuming, then, emotions aside, once and for all, to the satisfaction of everyone, that the cause turns out to be what so many already suspect it to be — exposure to chemicals in the environment — then what? With infectious disease, the idea is to prevent the problem by removing its source (eradicating mosquitoes to stop the spread of malaria, for example) or by neutralizing the impact of the disease agent (administering a vaccine against polio virus, say). But what in the world will anyone be able to do to prevent a disease caused by living in the twentieth century? Especially when the twentieth century has been defined by the impact of industrialization. What can we do about the noxious chemical effects of industrialization? Eradicate industry?

The notion is ridiculous (although there are more than a few who wouldn't mind seeing it happen). In lieu of that, however, what if it were possible to reorient industry? To make it desirable, *profitable*, to clean up its act. For Kaye Kilburn, that is our last chance.

Kilburn is a professor of environmental science at the University of Southern California School of Medicine. He makes no bones about the magnitude of the MCS problem. "MCS patients are articulating what's happening to all of us. We know now that this problem is a big one, a bigger problem than AIDS, certainly. It's probably related to the cancer problem, which is also largely chemically induced, despite the efforts to make it genetic. So it's time to act. We must move this effort into another arena — not just the research arena, but the action arena.

"What this means is that we must change our priorities for industry. We've got to make a change toward a chemically free world that is profitable. There are numerous examples of chasing toxic materials out of the chemical stream and increasing its profitability. An important one occurred in Salt Lake City when I was a medical student. The local copper refinery determined that the sulfur dioxide in the air, which was polluting the Salt Lake Valley and even killing trees and dairy cattle, could be removed by distilling it into water and making sulfuric acid. That not only had the enormous social benefit of reducing the sulfur dioxide in the entire Salt Lake Valley, but selling the product *paid* for the removal. It was *profitable.* So it is a matter of a change in priority. Often it can be profitable."

But, if such a change is even possible, it won't be easy, profitable or no. "We've grown up in a chemical world," Kilburn says. "So it's not conceivable to us that it's dangerous. It's like mistrusting our home. And having lived through the entire campaign against cigarette smoking, I realize how tough it can be. If we think that the tobacco companies fight hard and can be vicious, add up all the petrochemical companies and chemical production and you're looking at a far more gigantic goliath.

"But the battle against the tobacco companies offers more hope than anything else that we can do something about chemicals, despite far greater complexity and far larger targets. People finally were convinced to rise up and say, 'We want smoke-free environments.' And this went from being a small, vocal minority to being a majority."

Kilburn even sees glimmers of hope within the chemical industry itself. Pure self-interest may drive a reorientation to cleaner production. "Some individuals in positions of power, they realize the problem. I've seen instances when anti-MCS litigation was stopped because there was also a threat to stop treatment of families of chemical executives who were damaged by chemicals."

Al Levin also sees signs of change within the industry. "It's really kind of funny because these people are chasing their tails. For example, among the people in Dow Chemical Company who claim that Bill Rea is a quack, many of them go to him. Board chairmen go to him because they're sick. They know MCS exists, but it's not good for business. We're gonna make it good for business."

How? Through litigation. For Levin, that's the key. It's through litigation that he sees the chemical industries being *forced* to clean up their act. "People with MCS are canaries in the mine, definitely. But I don't think we are at a stage where we have poisoned our environment badly enough that it's irreversible. We used to use X-ray fluoroscopy to see if our shoes fit. Tell that to your kid and he'd say you're nuts. Well, we use a thousandfold more X rays today than we did in those days, but we're much more careful about it. Same thing about chemicals and pesticides. For instance, if we sprayed pesticides from the ground, and used metered amounts, we'd be fine. I'm gonna tell a ten-year-old boy in ten years that we used to spray pesticides from airplanes, and he'll have the same reaction: 'You can't be that dumb. Those are poisons!' We don't want to shut the companies down. We don't have to stop using these chemicals. We just have to stop being cavalier about it."

But, like Kilburn, Levin knows the fight is going to be tough. "The companies don't want to change. And there's so much money in lawsuits, the defense attorneys don't want the companies to change. We were suing one of the very large chemical corporations in this country about trichlorethylene in the water causing leukemia. In the last six months of the case the corporation was paying the defense firm a million dollars a month in fees — and two hundred thousand a month was going back to the executives of the corporations as expert consultants. So, yes, some people in the corporations are making money on the lawsuits, too."

But tough is the way Levin likes it. He is champing at the bit to use the litigation process to effect the kind of change he wants. "I have never seen a vehicle of social change that works as fast and effectively as the toxic tort arena. Never! And the toxic chemical lawsuits have done more for humanity than anything else. The bigger the settlement, the better it is. Let me tell you this: We are wearing safety belts in automobiles not because someone published in the *New England Journal of Medicine* but because somebody kicked somebody's tail in a lawsuit. That's the only way to get people to turn around — you have to hit 'em where they live, you have to cost 'em money. So these lawsuits are wonderful things. And the more money that is generated from them, the better it is for humanity."

Levin has now opened law offices in both Texas and California. He's hooked up with partners who share his vision, and his dissatisfaction, and his perilous background. "My new firm is made up of five old marines. San Francisco– and Houston-based. A lot of money behind it. A lot of guys that just don't give a shit and want to get the point across. It's a multipronged attack. The others are the Eisenhowers, MacArthurs — the accepted people. I'm the scum bucket, the black sheep. I'm the commando.

"I want Bill Rea to be my expert witness. We're gonna reform American industry and medicine. There are certain people that I've already lined up to file criminal charges against. The difference between me and other attorneys is that I will hold people to their oaths and I will attempt to get people for perjury.

I know I won't be successful in most cases, but I will make enough trouble that these people won't want to lie on the stand anymore. I'm gonna be on the phone with the attorney general every twenty minutes asking about the progress of the case. I'll make such a pest of myself that people are gonna have to investigate what I'm talking about. And some people are gonna fall hard, real hard. Some are gonna go to jail, end up selling shoes."

Levin pauses for a breath, a wicked gleam in his eyes. "My plan is to create a lot of havoc and make a lot of money."

It may be that the canaries are singing loudly enough after all. Their voices are growing harsher, more strident, more confident. As though they realize that they can no longer be ignored. As though they refuse to be ignored. And they're now singing out of the depths of Desert Storm as well as from the polluted buildings and streets of America. They're now singing in male voices as well as female, in young voices as well as old.

And more of them are singing. Whether from a heightened realization of their plight or simply because more and more people are becoming allergic to the twentieth century, no one knows. But the suspicion is growing that we're all in this together. Many of those who have seen their lives severely altered by MCS were once "normal," just like the rest of us. The many more less seriously afflicted try as best they can to live day to day, just like the rest of us. It may be that there is no 'rest of us.' And it may be that any of us, at any time, might find our own lives shattered because of our polluted environment.

Those who suffer multiple chemical sensitivity, those who treat it, those who have no doubt of its reality even if they can't yet put a finger on its cause, all those sense that something important is developing, a tidal wave of dissatisfaction and an insistence on finding answers. It may be no accident that just as chemical sensitivity is becoming a widespread health problem, public concern for a healthy environment is growing. What these pioneers discover will have powerful repercussions.

Says Al Levin, "We're in the Model T stage of this thing, really, really very crude. We're just beginning to see the tip of the iceberg."

MCS Resources[*]

• MCS Support Groups

Human Ecology Action League (HEAL)
PO Box 49126
Atlanta, GA 30359
404-248-1898

Chemical Injury Information Network (CIIN)
PO Box 301
White Sulphur Springs, MT 59645-0301
406-547-2255

National Center for Environmental Health Strategies (NCEHS)
1100 Rural Avenue
Voorhees, NJ 08043
609-429-5358

Environmental Health Advocacy League (ENHALE)
Box 425
Concord, MA 01742
508-287-4543

MCS Referral & Resources
2326 Pickwick Road
Baltimore, MD 21207
410-448-3319

---

* Most of these resources were recommended by people who suffer from multiple chemical sensitivity and Gulf War syndrome. I have no firsthand knowledge of many of them. Special thanks to Rick Kiessig, April Lang, and Erika Lundholm.

• Books

Ashford, Nicholas A., and Claudia S. Miller. *Chemical Exposures: Low Levels and High Stakes.* Van Nostrand Reinhold, 1991.

Bell, Iris R. *Clinical Ecology: A New Medical Approach to Environmental Illness.* Common Knowledge, 1982.

Dadd, Debra Lynn. *Nontoxic, Natural and Earthwise: How to Protect Yourself and Your Family from Harmful Products and Live in Harmony with the Earth.* J. P. Tarcher, 1990.

Krohn, Jacqueline. *The Whole Way to Allergy Relief and Prevention: A Doctor's Complete Guide to Treatment and Self-Care.* Hartley and Marks, 1996.

Lawson, Lynn. *Staying Well in a Toxic World: Understanding Environmental Illness, Multiple Chemical Sensitivities, and Sick Building Syndrome.* Noble Press, 1994.

Randolph, Theron G. *Environmental Medicine — Beginnings and Bibliographies of Clinical Ecology.* Clinical Ecology Publications, 1987.

Randolph, Theron G., and Ralph W. Moss. *An Alternative Approach to Allergies: The New Field of Clinical Ecology Unravels the Environmental Causes of Mental and Physical Ills.* HarperCollins, 1990.

Rapp, Doris. *Is This Your Child?: Discovering and Treating Unrecognized Food Allergies.* Morrow, 1991.

Rea, William J. *Chemical Sensitivity.* 4 vols. Lewis Publishers, 1992–1996.

Rogers, Sherry A. *Tired or Toxic?* Prestige, 1990.

Tate, Nicholas. *The Sick Building Syndrome: How Indoor Air Pollution Is Poisoning Your Life and What You Can Do.* New Horizon, 1993.

Upton, Arthur C., and Eden Graber, eds. *The New York University Medical Center Family Guide to Staying Healthy in a Risky Environment.* Simon & Schuster, 1993.

• Consultants

• *Chemical and Allergen Environmental Levels*

Mark Sneller
PO Box 575
Tucson, AZ 85702
520-326-4771
800-350-7129

• *Healthy Home Building*

Rick Kiessig
888 Nancy Lane
Los Altos, CA 94024
415-962-1705

• Supplies

• *Miscellaneous Supplies*

American Environmental Health Foundation
8345 Walnut Hill Circle
Suite 200
Dallas, TX 75231
800-428-2343
(air filters, nutritional supplements, water filters, bare metal beds, masks, shampoos, ceramic oxygen masks, etc.)

NEEDS
527 Charles Avenue
Suite 12A
Syracuse, NY 13209
800-634-1380
(health foods, nutritional supplements, books, air filters, shampoos, cosmetics, etc.)

• *Miscellaneous "Green" Supplies*

Living Source
3500 MacArthur Drive
Waco, TX 76708
817-756-6341

Real Goods
555 Leslie Street
Ukiah, CA 95482
800-762-7325
http://www.realgoods.com
realgood@realgoods.com

Seventh Generation
49 Hercules Drive
Colchester, VT 05446
800-456-1177

• *Cotton Beds and Clothing*

The Cotton Place
PO Box 59721
Dallas, TX 75229
800-451-8866
214-243-4149

Janice Corporation
198 Route 46
Budd Lake, NJ 07828
800-JANICES

Vermont Country Store
PO Box 3000
Manchester Center, VT 05255
800-362-4647

- *Cotton Futons and Poplar Futon Frames*

  Dona Designs
  825 Northlake Drive
  Richardson, TX 75080

- *Cotton Pillows*

  KB Cotton Pillows
  PO Box 57
  De Soto, TX 75115

- *Cotton Bedding, Futons, and Air Filters*

  Allergy Relief Shop
  2932 Middlebrook Pike
  Knoxville, TN 37921
  800-678-2028

- **Gulf War Veteran Organizations and Contacts**

- *Alabama*

  Gulf War Vets of Alabama, Inc.
  Contact: Dan Reeves
  2344 Glendale Avenue
  Montgomery, AL 36107
  Voice: 205-265-7723
  E-mail: 76163,1323@compuserve.com

- *Alaska*

  Desert Storm Justice Foundation — Alaska
  HC 89, Box 93
  Willow, AK 99688
  907-495-1205
  Fax: 907-495-1206

• *Arkansas*

  Gulf War Veterans of Arkansas
  Contact: Jeff Beer
  PO Box 1480
  Fairfield Bay, AR 72088
  Voice: 501-884-6352
  Fax: 501-884-6277
  E-mail: Jeff@gulfwar.org

• *California*

  California Association of Persian Gulf Veterans
  Contact: Erika Lundholm
  PO Box 3661
  Santa Cruz, CA 95063
  Voice: 408-476-6684
  Fax: 408-476-2847
  E-mail: lundholm@cruzio.com

  Northern California Association of Persian Gulf Veterans
  Contact: Debbie Judd
  9141 E. Stockton Boulevard
  #250-168
  Elk Grove, CA 95624
  Voice: 916-684-1693
  Fax: 916-684-1693
  E-mail: NCAPGV@aol.com

  Persian Gulf War Veterans Association of America
  Contact: Duane Mowrer
  Midvale Avenue
  Oakland, CA 94602
  Voice: 510-482-4931
  Fax: 510-530-6337
  E-mail: pgwva@aol.com

  Swords to Plowshares
  Contact: Dan Fahey
  995 Market Street, 3rd Floor

San Francisco, CA 94103
Voice: 415-247-8777
Fax: 415-227-0848

- *Colorado*

Desert Storm Veterans of the Rocky Mountains
Contact: Denise Nichols
4050 Cody
Wheat Ridge, CO 80033
Voice: 303-424-6235
Fax: 303-423-0437
E-mail: GJMF90B@prodigy.com

- *Connecticut*

Vietnam Veterans Agent Orange Victims, Inc.
Contact: Scott Vanderhyden
PO Box 2465
Darien, CT 06820
Voice: 203-656-0003
Fax: 202-656-1957
E-mail: VVAOV@humanics.sprint.com

- *Delaware*

Gulf War Veterans of Delaware
Contact: Sonny Evers
1505 Dilworth Road
Wilmington, DE 19805
Voice: 302-998-6087
E-mail: Sonny68@aol.com

- *District of Columbia*

National Gulf War Resource Center
1224 M Street NW
Washington, DC 20005
Voice: 202-628-2700, ext. 162
Fax: 202-628-6997
E-mail: Charles@gulfwar.org

- *Florida*

  Desert Storm Justice Foundation — Florida
  Contact: Bill Carpenter
  10 Marlow Road
  Frostproof, FL 33843-9321
  Voice: 813-635-3261
  E-mail: BillCarpenter@cjewel.com

  Desert Storm Veterans of Florida, Inc.
  Contact: Kevin Knight
  PO Box 6081
  Titusville, FL 32782
  Voice: 407-269-3453
  E-mail: GULFVET@metrolink.net

- *Georgia*

  Gulf War Veterans of Georgia, Inc.
  Contact: Paul Sullivan
  PO Box 823
  Decatur, GA 30030
  Voice: 404-377-3741
  Fax: 404-377-8789
  E-mail: 70711,3174@compuserve.com

- *Idaho*

  Desert Storm Justice Foundation — Idaho
  Contact: David and Debbie Smith
  3226 — 8th Street, #D
  Lewiston, ID 83501
  Voice: 208-798-0348

- *Indiana*

  Gulf Veterans International, Inc.
  Contact: Richard Haines
  4247 Valley Terrace
  New Haven, IN 47150
  Voice: 812-948-9366

- *Louisiana*

  Mission Project
  Contact: Tony Picou
  PO Box 92574
  Lafayette, LA 70509
  E-mail: missionproject@popalex1.linknet.net

- *Massachusetts*

  Persian Gulf Era Veterans, Inc.
  Contact: Steve Reynolds
  467 East Street
  Westwood, MA 02090
  Voice: 617-329-8149
  E-mail: rdmac@acs.bu.edu

- *Michigan*

  International Advocacy for Gulf War Syndrome
  Contact: Brian and Kim Martin
  2297 Westfield Drive
  Niles, MI 49107
  Voice: 616-684-5903
  E-mail: DSVETERAN@aol.com

- *Minnesota*

  Desert Storm Justice Foundation — Minnesota
  PO Box 186
  Buhl, MN 55713
  Voice: 218-258-3685

- *Missouri*

  Desert Storm Justice Foundation — Missouri
  Contact: Jim Brown
  PO Box 373
  Hannibal, MO 63401
  Voice: 314-248-0406

• *New York*

Gulf War Vets of Long Island
Contact: Jackie Olsen
100 Robinson
E. Patchogue, NY 11772
Voice: 516-289-1580
E-mail: DStormMom@aol.com

Persian Gulf Veterans of Upstate New York
418 Den Wit Terrace
PO Box 578
Canasota, NY 13032
Voice: 315-697-7513

Persian Gulf Veterans, Inc.
Contact: Beverly Place
212 Garfield Avenue
E. Rochester, NY 14445
Voice: 716-385-4097
Fax: 716-248-9896

• *North Carolina*

Desert Storm Veterans of North Carolina, Inc.
Contact: Kevin Treiber
11961 UNGC Station
Greensboro, NC 27412
Voice: 910-334-2627
Fax: 910-334-2627
E-mail: kptreibe@uncg.edu

Gulf War Veterans of North Carolina
Contact: Pat Finney
50 Carolina Shores Parkway
Calabash, NC 28467
E-mail: patfinn@aol.com

• *Ohio*

Gulf War Veterans of Ohio
620 Lake Avenue
Ashtabula, OH 44004

Veterans and Families Support Network — National
Contact: Gina Brown
5488 State Route 7
New Waterford, OH 44445
Voice: 216-457-0641
E-mail: VFSN@delphi.com

Veterans and Families Support Network — Ohio
Contact: Nan Corple
16298 Irish Ridge Road
Calcutta, OH 43920
Voice: 216-385-2705
E-mail: VFSN@delphi.com

Persian Gulf Veterans of W. Penn/W. Virginia/NE Ohio
Contact: Barry Walker
600 N. Market Street
East Palestine, OH 44413
Voice: 216-426-3202/3203
Fax: 216-426-3309

• *Oklahoma*

Desert Storm Justice Foundation — National
Contact: Gina Whitcomb
PO Box 16182
Oklahoma City, OK 73113
Voice: 405-348-1722
Fax: 405-348-8547
E-mail: dsjf@telepath.com

• *Oregon*

Northwest Veterans for Peace
Contact: Marvin Simmons
811 E. Burnside Street #218
Portland, OR 97214
Voice: 503-234-6242
E-mail: NWVP@teleport.com

• *South Carolina*

Persian Gulf War Veterans Association
245 Piney Grove Road
Columbia, SC 29210
Voice: 803-722-8615

Gulf War Veterans of the Carolinas
895 Eastwood Drive
Rock Hill, SC 29730
Voice: 803-328-0410

• *Tennessee*

American Gulf War Veterans
PO Box 78426
Nashville, TN 37207
Voice: 615-753-5336

Mountain Home Veterans Support Group
509 Meadow Brook Avenue
Jonesboro, TN 37659
Voice: 615-753-5336

Persian Gulf Information Network, Inc.
Contact: Paul Lyons
PO Box 10160
Clarksville, TN 37042
Voice: 615-431-5222
E-mail: PerGulf@aol.com

• *Texas*

Desert Storm Veterans Coalition
Contact: Betty Zuspann
PO Box 2313
Hewitt, TX 76643
Voice: 800-307-1330, 817-666-0489

Operation Desert Shield/Desert Storm Association (ODSA)
Contact: Vic Sylvester
PO Box 1712
Odessa, TX 79760
Voice: 915-368-4667
Fax: 915-368-4667
E-mail: 102753.3412@compuserve.com

Persian Gulf Veterans of America
Contact: Kathy Hughes
PO Box 190222
San Antonio, TX 78280
Voice: 210-666-4409
E-mail: KathyPGVA@aol.com

- *Vermont*

   Desert Storm Justice Foundation — Vermont
   Contact: Gerald Patch
   81 Olive Street
   Springfield, VT 05156
   Voice: 802-885-5403
   Fax: 802-885-2030

- *Virginia*

   Desert Storm Justice Foundation — Virginia
   Contact: Diane St. Julian
   PO Box 6812
   Alexandria, VA 22309
   Voice: 703-550-3943
   Fax: 703-550-1346

- *Wisconsin*

   Contact: Chris Kornkven
   419 South Washington Street
   Watertown, WI 53094
   Voice: 414-206-0562
   Fax: 414-206-0563
   E-mail: Kornkven@globaldialog.com

- *United Kingdom*

  Trauma After Care Trust
  Contact: Doug Morris
  Buttsfields, The Farthings
  Withington, Glos. GL54-4DF
  Voice: 011-44-142-289-0306
  Fax: 011-44-142-289-0498
  E-mail: tact@tacthq.demon.co.uk

  National Gulf War Veterans and Families Association
  Highgate Rappax Road
  Hale, Cheshire W A 150NR
  Voice: 011-44-161-980-7091
  E-mail: 100674.552@compuserve.com

  The Gulf Veterans Association
  MEA House
  5th Floor
  Ellison Place
  Newcastle Upon Tyne, NE1 8XS

- *Gulf War Syndrome Websites:*

  Desert Storm Justice Foundation: www.dsjf.org

  Gulf War Veterans of Arkansas: www.gulfwar.org/GWVA/

  Gulf War Veterans Resource Pages: www.gulfwar.org

  National Gulf War Resource Center, Inc.:
  www.gulfwar.org/Resource_Center

  Presidential Advisory Committee on Gulf War Veterans' Illnesses
  Home Page: www.gwvi.gov

  DOD GulfLink: www.dtic.dla.mil/gulflink

Index

Abou-Donia, Mohamed, 225, 226, 227
acetylcholine, 159, 160, 161
acetylcholine esterase (AChE), 226, 227
adaptation (masking), 103–4, 128, 164–65, 166
advertising: chemical-free products, 175–79; pharmaceutical drugs, 196
Agency for Toxic Substances and Disease Registry, 173
Agent Orange, 148–49, 205
AIDS, 149, 150, 162, 240
air-filtration systems, 36
air pollution, 77
allergies, 3–4; acquired sensitization, 60, 77–78; and cancer, 69–70; chemicals and, 77–78, 124, 153; definitions of, 58, 70–71; desert environment and, 38; environmental medicine and, 78–79, 88; and expulsion of toxins, 67–70; immune system response, 61–62, 71–72; MCS and, 58, 70, 72; medical study of, 58–59; parasitic worms and, 63–67, 69; testing for, 4, 87, 88–89, 101–2
allergists, 58, 71, 72, 78–79, 87, 147, 193
allergy shots, 62, 72, 87–88
allopathy, 194, 195
American Academy of Allergy and Immunology, 38–39, 127, 131
American Academy of Environmental Medicine (AAEM), 74, 79
American College of Allergy and Immunology, 74
American College of Physicians, 131
American Medical Association (AMA), 131; on MCS, 15, 113; and medical education, 194, 195
ammines, 238
anaphylactic shock, 4, 62
anaphylaxis, 60
animal dander, 68
animal experiments, 156, 161
anthrax, 71; vaccine, 215
antibodies, 60–61, 151
antihistamines, 62
apoptosis, 150
arthro-myo-neuropathy syndrome, 228
Ashford, Nicholas A., 172–73
Ashland Chemical, Inc., 190
asthma, 3, 62, 72, 126
autoimmune disease, 150, 151, 152
autointoxication, 119, 120
avoidance therapy, 83, 112
Axelrod, Patricia, 215

Barnes, Nora, 75–78
Bascom, Rebecca, 152, 153, 154–55
BASF Corporation, 190
B cells, 149, 151
Bell, Iris R., 155, 156–58
Benjamin Moore & Company, 185, 190
biological weapons, 214
birth control pills, 126
Black, Donald, 114, 131, 134–35
Bleckman, Barbara, 40, 41, 43–44
blood clotting, 81–82
blood enzymes, 226
Bloom, Lee, 37, 39, 40–41, 42, 43
botulism vaccine, 215